consultation
with a
plastic
surgeon

consultation with a

plastic surgeon

Ralph Leslie Dicker, M.D.
Victor Royce Syracuse, M.D.

Nelson-Hall, Chicago nh

Library of Congress Cataloging in Publication Data

Dicker, Ralph Leslie.
        Consultation with a plastic surgeon.

        Includes index.
        1. Surgery, Plastic. I. Syracuse, Victor Royce,
joint author. II. Title.
RD118.D5   617'.95   74-30176
ISBN 0-88229-201-3

Manufactured in the United States of America

contents

preface

This question and answer book is based on actual consultations patients have had with us and with other practicing plastic surgeons over a number of years. Our hope is to reach and to reassure the many people who are curious about cosmetic surgery but who are, for one reason or another, reluctant to take the step of seeking a consultation with a plastic surgeon. We realize that for some people even a decision to consult with a surgeon is a momentous one, and we know full well the fears inhibiting the average person contemplating this type of surgery.

Even after a patient has made an appointment with a plastic surgeon, his anticipation of encountering the surgeon becomes magnified in his mind and his tension builds with each passing day. The climax is reached when the patient passes through the portals of the surgeon's reception room.

Seeing other people who are seeking similar advice and recommendations should relax the patient. However, at this point, he may be thinking only about his personal reason for this visit, the hope that his real or fancied cosmetic abnormalities can be corrected. Only occasionally does he wonder what corrections the other patients in the room are seeking.

The patient having a consultation with a plastic surgeon differs from the patient seeking consultation with other physicians in one critical way: our patient visits the surgeon hoping he can *obtain* surgical correction; the other patient hopes he will *not* require surgical correction.

Finally, the moment of confrontation arrives, and the patient finds himself face to face with his plastic surgeon. The patient's preconceived ideas of the appearance and manners of the surgeon may be completely different from those he now sees. Regardless, patient and surgeon must establish a rapport in order to derive the most from this first visit.

The consultation begins with the patient stating his complaint. (The patient should never expect or fear that the surgeon will take the initiative in pointing out any cosmetic irregularity that he may notice.) The discussion that follows will be frank, lucid, intimate, and respectful. The successful encounter leaves the patient with a feeling of confidence in the judgment he receives from the surgeon.

Credentials and qualification may be checked before an appointment is made. The capable plastic surgeon sought for consultation is one who has been trained by one of two methods. He will have specialized basically in head and neck surgery and have additional training in cosmetic plastic surgery, or his discipline will be general plastic surgery and he will have additional instruction in cosmetic plastic surgery. Some plastic surgeons, particularly those trained in head and neck surgery, perform mainly cosmetic *facial* plastic surgery. In all cases the surgeons must have had *special* training in the field of cosmetic plastic surgery.

The well-trained cosmetic plastic surgeon will have certification in one of the following specialties: the head and neck surgeon is certified as a Diplomate of the American Board of Otolaryngology; the general plastic surgeon is certified by the American Board of Plastic Surgery; and eye surgeons, who are oculoplastic surgeons trained in cosmetic eyelid surgery, are certified by the American Board of Ophthalmology. The head and neck surgeon trained in performing cosmetic surgery is usually a member of the American Academy of Facial Plastic and Reconstructive Surgery. The general surgeon or plastic surgeon trained in performing cosmetic surgery will usually be a member of the American Society of Plastic Surgeons. The eye surgeon trained in cosmetic eyelid surgery will usually be a member of the American Society of Oculoplastic and Reconstructive Surgery.

To choose your cosmetic plastic surgeon you may inquire of your county medical society requesting the names of local surgeons trained in cosmetic plastic surgery or the address of the American Academy of Facial Plastic and Reconstructive Surgery or the American Society of Plastic and Reconstructive Surgery or the American Society of Oculoplastic and Reconstructive Surgery, and request that they provide you with the names of cosmetic plastic surgeons in your area. Your family physician may be able to recommend a qualified cosmetic plastic surgeon. Lastly, any friend who has had successful plastic surgery performed should be happy to give you the name of his or her plastic surgeon for consultation.

The consultation includes history taking and an examination by a surgeon. After examination, the surgeon gives the patient his diagnosis, opinion, and recommendation. If the surgery is recommended by the plastic surgeon, the period is now open for questions and answers. Medical questions will be answered by the surgeon; nonmedical questions will be answered by an experienced secretary or medical assistant.

If surgery is not recommended, the surgeon will state his reasons. Surgery may not be recommended for many medical reasons, such as uncontrollable diabetes or hypertension, or the presence of cancer or tuberculosis. A well-trained surgeon can usually determine on the initial visit if the patient is a good or poor medical risk.

Another primary reason for not recommending surgery will be the surgeon's estimate of the deformity as being too minor. The deformity may exist only in the mind of the patient. Patients have traveled half the world to visit a plastic surgeon only to be told that their conditions in no way warrant plastic surgical procedures. Such patients may need evaluation by a psychiatrist who would try to help them to understand their neurosis about an imaginary defect.

If surgery is recommended and agreed upon by the patient, the surgeon will then arrange a future booking date, with the secretarial staff taking over the details of hospital arrangements, fees, insurance coverage, and all other nonmedical problems.

Through the question and answer format of this book we hope to portray the intimate phase of the consultation. We have used patients' questions and surgeons' answers, re-phrasing them occasionally so they may be more easily understood. The questions patients ask plastic surgeons fall into recognizable patterns, so much so that we think this book represents the accumulated experience of plastic surgeons in consultation with patients. Surgeons, like other craftsmen, belong to organizations, academies, and societies established for the exchange of ideas and experiences. Through their free flowing discussion with colleagues, surgeons learn what information patients are seeking. Such questions are answered in the chapters ahead. For this reason, we feel this book will be a source of ready information on the broad subject of cosmetic plastic surgery.

We believe there is hardly a person who is not interested in self-improvement. Even the person who is satisfied to live with a gross deformity may appreciate learning facts concerning his deformity. There are individuals who develop a placid demeanor which masks a deep disturbance over a cosmetic deformity. Actually, these people are fearful of surgery and assume an air of acceptance of their abnormalities. This book will permit them to search out the answers to their questions in privacy and will encourage a more realistic attitude to their problem. Fears and embarrassment will no longer prevent their becoming knowledgeable about this subject.

We have covered in this book vital questions about discomforts encountered in surgery, length of hospitalization and disability, time required away from employment, possibility of complications, degree of improvement anticipated, surgical fees, anesthesia requirements, and many other important subjects that arise in consultation. Whenever possible we have refrained from extensive use of technical words in order to make the answers to the patients' questions readily understandable. Terminology not routinely used in consultation is defined in the glossary.

While discussing words, we will make a brief foray into the semantics of this surgical specialty by pointing out the synonymous use of words like "cosmetic" plastic surgery and "aesthetic" plastic surgery. These words are used to describe a corrective plastic surgical procedure which aims to restore normal features and functions ("normal" means according to average standards of size, contour, and motion). Earlier in the Preface, we used the words "facial" plastic surgery and "general" plastic surgery. Facial plastic surgery includes cosmetic (or aesthetic) and reconstructive surgery of the face. General plastic surgery includes facial and body surgery, both cosmetic (or aesthetic) and reconstructive.

Reconstructive surgery of the face refers to surgery performed for congenital and acquired defects. Congenital abnormalities include cleft palate, harelip, and the absence of facial features at birth. Acquired defects are those due to traumatic injuries that destroy facial features. Reconstructive surgery of the face is also performed to correct abnormalities arising from disease, such as cancer, tuberculosis, or leprosy, which can destroy the nose or ears or large portions of the face.

Reconstructive surgery of the body refers to surgery for congenital defects, such as missing fingers or toes; surgery to correct portions of the body destroyed by injury, disease or previous surgery, such as radical mastectomy.

Cosmetic or aesthetic surgery refers to surgery for improvement of the artistic and natural beauty of the face or body. Within this category of surgical correction are face lift, nasal reconstruction, eyelid surgery, external ear surgery, breast augmentation or reduction, excision of facial and body scars, dermal abrasion for acne scars, hair transplantation, and body surgery for excessive skin and fatty tissue of the abdomen, thighs, or buttocks.

We have devoted our attention in this book to the questions and answers arising in consultation in the field of cosmetic or aesthetic plastic surgery.

We dedicate our book to our colleagues and instructors in the field of cosmetic plastic surgery whose efforts at meetings, in courses, in personal instruction and publications have contributed to the degree of excellence achieved in this specialty. The surgeon does not pull himself up by his own bootstraps. He is a finely honed product of the genius and tender loving care of his mentors.

For many years we have had the good fortune to be exposed to the exciting exchange of ideas at national and international meetings and congresses. At these meetings every skill of cosmetic plastic surgery and its results are explored, discussed in conference, described in lectures, and demonstrated by films and slides.

Organizations which have earned great respect for devotion to the development and progress in the field of cosmetic plastic surgery are the prestigious American Academy of Facial Plastic and Reconstructive Surgery, the American Society of Plastic and Reconstructive Surgery, and the American Academy of Ophthalmology and Otolaryngology. We, like all other cosmetic plastic surgeons, owe thanks to the many men in these organizations who from the beginning have taken the time to unselfishly pass along their knowledge and experience for the benefit of others in their field.

the modern history of plastic surgery

*We restore, repair, and make whole
parts which nature hath given, but
which fortune hath taken away.*

Gaspare Tagliacozzi
Father of Plastic Surgery
1597

The First World War (1914-1918) attracted the world's attention to plastic surgery. That new and revolutionary sort of war, fought by armies of millions, produced the inevitable thousands of casualties. Their injuries were often of a ghastly nature never experienced before. Although many more lives were saved than in previous wars, severely wounded soldiers were left with hideous deformities. Through the ingenuity and genius of military surgeons, many of these war victims were rescued. Modern plastic surgery, born out of the travail of this devastating war, succeeded in the herculean task of surgical rehabilitation through reconstruction of the deformed face and body.

With the end of the war in 1918, the conditions which had encouraged this great advance into the scientific specialty of plastic surgery appeared to vanish. However, with the spread of highway motoring at great speeds peacetime casualties were presenting an ever-increasing number of severe injuries and resultant deformities. In factories, the use of machines and mass-production methods and the employment of thousands of semi-skilled and unskilled workers increased the injuries requiring rehabilitative surgery.

At the beginning of the Second World War in the United States (1941) and in Great Britain (1939), the basic importance of plastic surgery was recognized from the start. The modern military surgeon was taught plastic surgical techniques and principles as the basis of the treatment of war casualties. The aim was restoration of function and the improvement of appearance. No casualty was considered fit for discharge until all that could possibly be done to restore his normal appearance, as well as normal function, had been carried out.

More than anything else, a number of great discoveries made possible the splendid surgical achievements of the war years, namely the discovery and introduction of the sulfa drugs and then—still more valuable—penicillin. These drugs enabled the surgeon to proceed with long and complicated surgical procedures with the assurance that infection, the deadly enemy of all good surgery, could be controlled.

A new technique enabled the plastic surgeon to turn these developments to striking uses. With fine, uniform, evenly cut sheets of skin made available by the new surgical dermatome, and the area of the defect clear of infection due to antibiotics, the grafting of extensive areas of skin was undertaken.

In World War I a high proportion of casualties succumbed to shock from burns or wounds. The availability of blood plasma in considerable quantities and the development of dried plasma revolutionized the treatment of shock.

When the patient was sufficiently recovered from shock, the plastic surgeon took over the plastic repair and reconstruction of the injured part. The tubed pedical graft, introduced in the First World War, began to be used more extensively for skin replacement, especially so because antibiotics were at hand to combat any signs of infection. One of the most notable of these techniques was the use of the delayed skin flaps with two or more migrations of the flap toward the site to be reconstructed.

Lastly, in recent years the public has become aware that a large percentage of deformities can be minimized or eliminated, especially in the aging process, to maintain a more attractive personal appearance with the aid of cosmetic surgery. The pressing demands for this surgery have found expression in a vast number of contributions from research and experimentation of surgeons in many countries.

There is no clear separation between the surgery of injury, plastic repair, and cosmetic surgery. The plastic surgeon must be conversant with all three. It may be fairly said, however, that while the reconstructive surgeon is more concerned with restoration of function, the cosmetic plastic surgeon deals with operations designed to alter contour or remove aesthetic defects. He must plan this so that no scar is visible; or if that ideal cannot be achieved, he must place the incision in a fold, or somewhere in shadow so that the scar is detectable only on the closest inspection and so that the patient will suffer the least handicap in his business and social affairs.

Thus has cosmetic plastic surgery evolved as a true surgical specialty—one with all surgical procedures in its entrance into the body by scalpel and yet apart from all other surgical procedures in its goal of restoring youth, beauty, and normality of appearance.

section 1
face lift surgery

Diamonds may be a girl's best friend, but they lose their luster to the aging matron when she looks in the mirror. She is often tempted to trade in her diamonds for a new face. She frequently does. Despite the counterculture rumblings telling us to "let it all hang out," women recognize all too clearly that we are fast becoming a youth-dominated society.

The male may have obtained great prominence in his field and accumulated great wealth in bank accounts, but he too may feel insecure when he views himself in the mirror and sees the lines deepening as each year passes. Because the male does not use the mirror with the frequent and penetrating study of the woman, his shock can be more devastating when he does stop long enough to look closely at his reflection. A man's greatest expression of his accomplishment is through his career, and it is fear of jeopardizing his future that sends chills down his spine at signs of aging. Increasing numbers of career oriented females are facing these same pressures because they must compete with youth in the business world as well as the social world.

With rejuvenation created by the plastic surgeon's face lift, there is a resurgence of physical activity, a renewed vigor in vocation, a revived interest in social contacts, and "another chance" for those whose happiness was abruptly threatened by the loss of a mate. Psychological stimulation is probably the explanation. If so, a few hours spent with a facial plastic surgeon are spent profitably in comparison to time spent in silent desperation.

Cosmetic plastic surgery is a remarkable method for eliminating most of the undesirable facial characteristics of the aging man or woman. The face lift can correct wrinkles of the cheek; the sagging of the skin into jowls which cause loss of the firm youthful outline of the lower jaw or mandible; the deepening of the groove of the outer nostril of the nose to the angle of the mouth; the groove from the angle of the mouth to the border of the lower jaw which creates a doughnut-circumoral pattern; the wrinkled skin that sags under the chin and forms cords from the chin down to the chest; and the folds of the "turkey gobbler" falling from the chin to mid-neck.

The surgical procedures to eliminate these undesirable manifestations of aging are adapted so that the telltale evidence of surgery, such as fine scars, are hidden within the hairline of the head above the ear and the natural fold in front and behind the ear and from behind the ear into the scalp above the hairline of the neck. This fine scar, when healed several weeks after surgery, is not noticeable to others.

Discomfort from the operative procedure is minimal since local anesthesia (the anesthesia of choice), preoperative medications, and the additive drugs administered during the operation combine to relax the patient and put him in a euphoric state. The majority of patients sleep deeply throughout the operation because of this method of anesthesia.

Some patients have a past history of experiencing pain with the use of local anesthesia and routine preoperative medications. They fear another such experience and request general anesthesia. The surgeon is not reluctant to give this particular patient general anesthesia; however, he knows that when the anesthetist administers general anesthesia he is not in favor of the surgeon's using agents such as adrenalin, at the operative site, for control of bleeding. The anesthetist fears the patient will develop cardiac irregularity or even cardiac arrest.

The surgeon explains to the patient that there may be more bleeding during and after the operation if general anesthesia is used. Therefore, in order to prevent accumulation of blood under the skin flaps, the surgeon using general anesthesia may insert rubber drains under the flaps for a short period postoperatively. If the bleeding is profuse, he will insert a hemovac (a suction apparatus) for one or two days postoperatively. The hemovac will not prevent the patient from ambulating during his hospital stay. The hospitalization could be one or two days longer for these patients.

When an operation is performed under local anesthesia, the bleeding during the operative procedure is well controlled and there is seldom a need for insertion of rubber drains or a hemovac. Patients can leave the hospital the morning after surgery. The total hospital stay is usually forty-eight to seventy-two hours.

If the patient has pain following the operative procedure, it can easily be controlled with pills such as Darvon Plain or Tylenol, medications slightly stronger than aspirin. Aspirin is to be avoided because experimentation has proven that bleeding is induced and is more copious when aspirin is taken following surgery. Detailed studies of aspirin taken after tonsillectomies have taught surgeons to avoid aspirin for postoperative patients for at least one week.

When the patient leaves the hospital, he is advised to avoid lifting heavy objects, to refrain from excessive bending or stretching, and to engage in only mild activity for a period of one week. Every effort is made to avoid postoperative bleeding and strain on the sutures holding the skin flaps together. If the patient has a sedentary position he may resume work immediately with a suitable hair covering—a wig for a man or a woman, or a kerchief for women. Normal activity can be resumed two weeks postoperatively. Those people who engage in strenuous muscular activity will require about three or four weeks of recovery before resuming such activities.

The surgeon attempts to remove sutures as early as possible (four to seven days) to avoid leaving suture marks. Some traction sutures which aid in elevating the facial muscles remain in place longer and are removed two weeks after the operation.

During this postoperative period the patient will experience a feeling of facial and cervical (neck) tightness and numbness. The analgesics mentioned earlier, Darvon Plain and Tylenol, are adequate for control of discomfort. At no time postoperatively is it necessary for patients to have a narcotic such as morphine or meperidine (Demerol) for pain.

Every plastic surgeon will explain preoperatively to the patient the improvement he may expect from the routine face lift operation. He will call attention to the fact that corrective eyelid surgery for wrinkles and fatty protrusions under the eyes (bagginess) are not a routine part of the face lift. Both procedures can be performed at the same time if the surgeon and the patient agree to this additional surgery. If the patient is not in good enough physical condition for an additional two hours of surgery on the eyelids, the surgeon will discourage him from undergoing both procedures in one surgical period. A complete face lift takes three to four hours, and the usual length of a combined operation of face lift and eyelids is four to six hours. Even if the patient is hardy enough for six hours of surgery, the surgeon may not be!

There are grooves and lines of the face, forehead, eyelids, and upper lip which cannot be removed with a routine face lift. Also heavy fat accumulations under the chin are not eliminated routinely. Additional surgical procedures must be resorted to in order to improve these areas. Fine lines and grooves will need chemo-surgery (acid, such as phenol formulas) or dermabrasion. The fat pads under the chin may require a special surgical procedure since it is surgically difficult to remove chin fat at the time of routine face lift. For chin fat pads a direct T-shaped incision under the chin is made and the fat and superfluous skin are removed. The sutures in the skin are under great stress when this procedure is performed with the routine face lift. Therefore, the procedure is best performed several months after the face lift.

A face lift will last five to ten years depending upon the age group of the patient, his normal activities, and his biological genes. The characteristics of the patient's skin, whether thick or thin, oily or dry, fair or dark complexioned, are important variants in determining the lasting quality of a face lift.

Fees for a face lift operation are $1,500 to $5,000 as quoted by plastic surgeons throughout the country. The average fee is $2,500.

It would be wonderful to contemplate the prospect of the face lift as the panacea for restoration of our youthful appearance. However, the face covers an area of about one-eighth of the entire body, so that beyond our neck we hide the further damaging evidence of aging. Today's surgeons are prepared to go beyond the face lift to return youthfulness to women by rejuvenating their bosoms, reducing pendulous abdomens, buttocks, thighs, and arms, inserting silicone experimentally into wrinkled, aged hands, and removing the brown spots and fatty skin infiltrations of aging on the face and body and hands.

Experiments with chemical injections are being performed to study methods of halting the aging of the skeletal structure and to prevent the insidious destruction of the aging brain by arteriosclerosis (hardening of the arteries of the brain). We await these discoveries with breathless anticipation just as we await the breakthrough in cancer diagnosis and therapy. Meanwhile nothing better can be offered for the scars of aging than cosmetic plastic surgery. The face lift is one of the most skillfully performed feats of the plastic surgeon.

Can a patient with a heart condition
safely have a face lift operation?

Your facial plastic surgeon will first require you to have a physical examination by your general doctor, internist, or cardiologist and will request that a written report of your present medical status be sent to him. The report should include an opinion as to whether or not you are a suitable candidate for surgery of this nature. If necessary, the plastic surgeon will discuss the risks of surgery with your doctor.

The adrenalin component of anesthetic agents increases both heartbeat and blood pressure. Limiting the proportion of adrenalin raises the probability of excessive bleeding. A patient using anticoagulants for postcoronary therapy may be discouraged from elective surgery unless the anticoagulant can be safely omitted for several days before surgery. This can be done only on the advice of a cardiologist, who would know if there is a risk of another coronary attack.

Many patients who have had heart and other medical problems have had successful facial plastic surgery because the surgeon was concerned with their total well-being.

Does high blood pressure contraindicate facial plastic surgery?

Facial surgery is not contraindicated because a patient is being treated for high blood pressure. Most facial plastic surgery is performed under local anesthesia, which interferes the least with the patient's condition of higher than normal blood pressure. However, before you enter the hospital the cosmetic surgeon will require you to be examined by your family physician or internist, who will provide a written report for the surgeon, testifying to the fact that all necessary measures are being taken to control the blood pressure and stating the patient is in sufficient good health to undergo surgery with local anesthesia. The patient may even be advised to spend two days in bed with proper sedation prior to surgery, a measure which greatly aids in lowering the blood pressure.

Can a man have a face lift despite loss of hair?

Sparsity of hair does not prevent a man from having face lift surgery. If he has sufficient temporal hair, incisions are made immediately above the ear, well within the hair of the temples, where baldness seldom occurs, and continue down and around behind the ear into the scalp hair. This approach permits the surgeon to do a complete revision of the facial skin and to lift the drooping eyebrow where necessary.

On men who have sparse temporal hair, as well as on those men who have no need of excision of excess skin in the forehead area, the procedure of choice will be an incision from the outer canthus (corner) of the eye to the superior pole of the ear. This type of incision is continued with the usual incision in front of the ear, under the lobe of the ear, and continues behind the ear to halfway up, then veers horizontally backward into the hair of the scalp. The fine scar that results from the outer corner of the eye to the ear heals well, having been finely and carefully sutured so as to produce a barely noticeable linear scar that gradually fades. During the healing process the scar is easily and entirely hidden from view by the temples of a pair of plastic eyeglass frames.

Will the wearing of dentures make any difference in having a face lift?

Wearing dentures will not interfere in any way with cosmetic face lift surgery. Dentures are worn to normalize the relation of the upper jaw to the lower jaw. If the dentures are fitted successfully, good dental occlusion should result and restore harmony to the facial features. When a face lift is performed, the patient is usually instructed to wear his dentures because local anesthesia is administered, enabling the surgeon to better gauge the extent of correction needed. If a patient is in the process of being fitted with dentures, he should postpone surgery until the dentures are satisfactorily fitted.

As a male I wonder how many men request face lift surgery. Are there any statistics to show the comparison of male and female requests?

The open discussion of face lift surgery by prominent men in public life has made people aware of the prevalence of this type of cosmetic surgery performed on males. It is estimated at this time that about 25 percent of the requests for cosmetic plastic surgery (face lifts and eyelid surgery) are from males. The publicity some men have had (and perhaps have given themselves) following facial plastic surgery also points up why face lifts (and blepharoplasties) are on the increase for the male. The public image—on stage, in the political forum, at the corporate director's meeting, or at a swinging cocktail party—is the driving force that sends men to the facial plastic surgeon. "I can't afford to look my age—let alone look old," a male patient said succinctly. He was referring to aging as a threat to his financial, political, and social position. The crux of the problem is that advancing age jeopardizes the male's position of power and prestige. He may feel being replaced by a younger man is to be avoided at all costs—and one of these costs is facial plastic surgery.

With the resurgence of confidence in his new appearance comes the "second wind" for the vigorous, middle-aged man. Suddenly he is imbued with great courage to face his competition. As facial plastic surgeons we have sent many older males back to the public arena to beat off the younger male animals.

How can I persuade my reluctant husband that I should have facial plastic surgery?

There may be urgent motives for your having aesthetic plastic surgery that deserve your trying some intelligent and gentle persuasion. You may have a career you are unwilling to relinquish and that is dependent upon your attractive youthful appearance. You may be suffering in silent desperation when you look at yourself in the mirror and see what aging has wrought. You may need a "whole new you" to shake off the "blues" of the menopause years. These are valid reasons for desiring cosmetic plastic surgery and these should be freely discussed with your husband. If he realizes your decision is not based on a whim but on a serious evaluation of your need for this improvement in your appearance, your husband may relent and respect your wishes. Put him in a good mood and verbalize your hidden desires to look younger (as long as they are not to attract another man!). If you do not succeed, you may have what some women might envy you for, "the perfect husband." He sees you as the young beauty he fell in love with and married for better or for worse.

Of course there are often valid reasons for a husband's objection to his wife's contemplating plastic surgery. There may be financial obligations that take precedence over the costs of this type of elective surgery. He may have strong feelings about not wanting any physical change in the appearance of a loved one. He may feel that a physical change could be followed by a personality change. Your husband may also harbor a fear of the risks that are inherent in all major surgery. He may be more willing to live with aesthetic imperfection than to run the risks of surgery.

I am divorced and am now dating a woman twenty years younger than myself. What can I do to make myself look younger?

The answer to your question is all in the mirror. Your eyelids need corrective surgery for the loose skin and "bagginess" under the lower eyelids. A face lift would eliminate or minimize the jowls and deep folds between your nose and mouth (nasolabial fold) and mouth and chin (paralabial fold), and draw up the pouchy, sagging skin beneath the chin. Your appearance would surely be that of a younger man, and if you follow a regimen of exercise and healthful diet for your age (high protein and low calorie), you will have a fighting chance to beat off the young swains. And then there is always the consolation that as your youthful appearance retrogresses, so will her aging process progress. She may need facial plastic surgery for the first time before you need it for the second time!

Will health insurance coverage pay for a face lift? Will Medicare make any allowance for a face lift?

Most health insurance plans have a clause excluding benefits for plastic surgery. Since the face lift operation is cosmetic plastic surgery, the exclusion clause would nullify surgical claims for a face lift procedure.

Cosmetic face lift surgery is sometimes performed in conjunction with the surgical treatment of conditions, such as partial paralysis of the muscles of the face, as in Bell's Palsy, or following mastoidectomy and surgery for parotid (salivary) tumors, benign or malignant, as well as for dermatological conditions. Where such complications exist, a full report of the diagnosis and surgical procedure from the surgeon to the insurance company will probably bring some allowance for benefits for both hospitalization and surgery.

Since the surgeon cannot be expected to review each patient's insurance program or to be qualified to interpret the fine print exclusion clauses, the patient who is concerned about insurance benefits should discuss this problem with the agent or company issuing the policy. Even the Blue Cross and Blue Shield plans, with which many surgeons are familiar, vary from state to state. A definitive answer about the benefits allowed by insurance plans should not be sought from the surgeon.

I have read of isometric exercises for the face. Would these be recommended for use before or after a face lift?

It has not been sufficiently established that so-called isometric exercises are useful before or after the face lift operation. We know that actors and actresses (whose talent depends upon the ability to portray the whole gamut of emotions through facial expressions) overuse their facial muscles to such a degree that their faces age earlier than they would ordinarily, showing wrinkles, furrows, and "smile" and "frown" lines. If it is possible to encourage wrinkling by overuse of muscles, there is well-grounded suspicion that isometric exercises may do more harm than good.

There are certain isometric exercises (based on forcing muscles to work against each other and against opposing surrounding tissue) that allegedly help to lift

the deep crevices of the nasolabial fold (nose to mouth),
the weakened muscles of the lower eyelids, and the
sagging muscles below the chin. The exercise itself
resembles a combination of blowing bubbles and forcing
the eyelids to a slitlike position. However, how frequently and for how long a period of time the exercises
should be practiced have not been established.

**Why is it that my upper lip has many
fine age lines whereas my husband, who
is my age, does not show this aging on
his lip? Would a face lift help rid
me of lip lines?**

The firm upper lip in the male is endowed with numerous tough hairs and hair follicles. His moustache is
embedded in a dense substratum of connective tissue
under thick skin. This kind of skin of the male upper lip
wrinkles with great difficulty, if at all. The female upper
lip, differently constructed and lacking the above elements of support, wrinkles easily, producing in time vertical furrows that are a disfiguring telltale of the aging
process.

The face lift is not the ideal solution to the problem
of vertical lip lines and furrows. Other courses of action
are more effective. Chemical peeling or dermal abrasion
is recommended instead. Either can be performed along
with the face lift or as a separate procedure.

**I have a double chin. Can it be corrected?
Is this a part of the face lift?**

The operation for the double chin, which is caused by a
fat pad, can be corrected with a submental lipectomy
(removal of extraneous fat and skin). The incision line
spans about one and a half inches in length just beneath
and behind the chin. Here is where the fat is removed
from under the skin. The ready access to the area and
the resultant youthful appearance following it warrant
having the double chin corrected by this incision, which

heals as a fine line hidden from direct view by the chin.

The surgery is most frequently performed separately, not in conjunction with the face lift, although this is certainly not a hard and fast rule with plastic surgeons. When an excess fatty pad continues to "hang there" under the chin after a face lift, it can be removed surgically after the complete healing of the face lift incisions.

There are mechanical devices being sold to stimulate electrically the muscles of the face. Would this device be helpful to use before or after a face lift operation?

Vibrating devices have been around for a long time in the field of physical health and beauty. There are enthusiastic advocates of this approach to body and face care. Medical opinion is extremely dubious about the degree of effectiveness of these products, except to acknowledge that any vibrating device, if used on a healthy person (and not *overused,* is often stimulating to one receiving the treatment, encouraging his feeling of well-being. It also increases the blood circulation in the skin layers at the points of contact. This too, like hand massage, may be of some small value.

That vibrating devices strengthen the weakened sagging muscles is questionable if not entirely improbable. In fact, excessive manipulation of the facial skin can rupture the fibers connecting the skin to the subcutaneous tissues, especially if done shortly after face lift surgery. No facial manipulation by hand or electrical device should be performed less than six months after facial surgery.

Where facial muscles show weakness or partial paralysis after face lift, stimulating electrical current, carefully calibrated for intensity, is beneficial.

How can I put myself in the right
frame of mind and overcome the fear I
have for a face lift operation?

To put yourself in the right frame of mind requires you to see yourself as others see you. Even looking at yourself in the mirror may not reveal all the truth about yourself. An untouched close-up photograph at a distance from your face of about three or four feet will reveal every defect that other people see on you. One look at these photographs (taken professionally, if possible) will convince you that you need surgery, or that you have exaggerated your condition in your mind.

If you have made a decision in favor of surgery, you then should choose a plastic surgeon for consultation concerning your facial deformities. If this step is an additional obstacle because of your fears, remember that facial plastic surgery has become as commonplace as any general surgery today and that you are merely consulting with a qualified specialist to confirm your decision for corrective facial surgery. The doctor will search out your desires for facial improvement and your fears about the surgery during consultation.

Have no hesitation in telling him your innermost thoughts on this vital experience in your life. He is well prepared for such a heart-to-heart talk, having known the fears and ultimate joy of others like yourself. If he concurs that facial surgery would give you the improved, more youthful appearance you desire, he will do all in his power to allay your fears and to gain your complete confidence.

If you have a specific dread of anesthesia and possible pain, you are reminded that no surgeon can perform an operation unless the patient is quiet and relaxed. This state of euphoric bravado is reached by administering to you suitable premedication.

Shortly before your hospital entrance day, you will

probably be prescribed a tranquilizer to relieve appre-
hension. When you are admitted as a patient to the
hospital, you will undergo a thorough physical examination and have laboratory tests to verify your good
health. You will begin to receive medications to prepare
you for a safe and comfortable operative procedure.

In the evening before surgery, you will receive a
capsule that will provide you with a good night's rest.
You will be awakened in the morning to receive another
capsule to continue your relaxation in preparation for
surgery. An injection will induce a twilight sleep, and
you will look forward to having this much-wanted plastic surgery with no trace of fear or hesitation. It will
amaze you to realize how fearless you have become with
surgery only minutes away.

**Is it best to have facial plastic
surgery in the winter or summer?**

There is nothing seasonal about facial plastic surgery.
Your surgeon works all year round; the hospitals are
prepared to perform their services January through
December; your face heals equally well in every season.
The factors involved in determining your choice of winter or summer are those only incidental to surgery:
When can you allow one or two weeks for personal
matters? If you are told to refrain from sunbathing, can
you abide by the instructions? When does your surgeon
take *his* vacation and consequently become unavailable
for surgery? Would you miss passing up winter or summer sports for a few weeks? Choose your time of surgery without concern for your ability to heal according
to the temperature outdoors.

If you are one who sneezes frequently during the
winter season due to chronic nasopharyngitis or upper
respiratory infections or one who sneezes frequently in
the spring and summer season due to allergens present
during those months of the year, avoid your vulnerable

sneezing months, if possible. However, seasonal sneezing at any time of the year, not associated with infection, can be controlled with antihistamines and permit facial plastic surgery to be performed throughout the year irrespective of season or climate.

What indicates to the surgeon that the male patient seeking face lift surgery has a completely reasonable and normal attitude to this surgery?

The male patient seeks face lift surgery in the proper frame of mind if he discusses his frank desire to look younger by eliminating *some* of the facial signs of aging. He desires to perform well in the socioeconomic sphere of life. *He expects no miracles.* He knows a younger looking face is no substitute for younger arteries.

Emotional disturbances in men are more subtle and deep rooted than in women. It takes more probing on the part of the surgeon to uncover psychoneuroses in the male, since the male has a greater capacity to cover up emotional and mental disturbances. If the surgeon sees signs of emotional instability that could jeopardize a normal attitude to a plastic surgical procedure, the surgeon will discourage the patient from seeking a cosmetic change in his appearance.

The mentally adjusted patient is one who would be able to accept jibes from his friends and relatives for having undergone plastic surgery. He must be able to accept a possible disappointment in the degree of cosmetic improvement attained if he does not look twenty years younger in the mirror.

Is the "morning after" look of fatigue actually due to a routine of late hours and hard work (or hard play), or is it a sign of aging?

Hard living and chronological aging are the combined enemies of the youthful appearance. There is no doubt that excessive debauching, heavy smoking, lack of sleep, overeating, excessive tension during long working hours, and too infrequent leisure hours are conducive to premature aging. Physiologically, the body muscles become fatigued and lose their normal tensile strength, like a worn out rubber band. Dramatic actors and actresses are known for the overuse of facial expressions in their work and thereby develop early wrinkling of the skin and sagging of the muscles. Arteriosclerosis, hypertension, and diabetes come earlier to those people who are self-indulgent in their diet and mode of living. Excessive smoking causes cancer and emphysema of the lungs with resultant respiratory difficulties. Excessive drinking of alcohol brings on cirrhosis of the liver and changes in the arteries that supply the heart and brain. Naturally all these internal changes are reflected externally in the skin and muscles of the face and body.

Can a person seventy or eighty years old have cosmetic surgery, in particular, a face lift?

The patient in his seventies or eighties daydreams of how attractive he was in his fifties and sixties. There is no doubt in his mind when he looks in the mirror that he appears elderly, and he finds his appearance distressing, even depressing. He wishes to restore some semblance of youth to his elderly face and seeks the aid of a plastic surgeon. When the plastic surgeon consults with this patient, his first thoughts are of the general health and mental condition of the patient. He asks the patient to give him a history of present and past complaints and known ailments.

The surgeon is interested in the answers to these questions:

Do you have a cardiac condition?
Do you have high blood pressure?
Do you bruise or bleed easily?
Do you have diabetes?

Do you take drugs for any medical condition?

Do you smoke excessively?

Do you exercise?

Why do you want plastic surgery?

The last question is important to determine the mental and emotional attitudes of the patient. The plastic surgeon does not want to perform cosmetic surgery on an elderly person who has a chronic illness or debilitating disease, nor does he want to operate on a senile, mentally disturbed individual. The surgeon must feel that the elderly patient can endure with safety three or four hours of surgery.

What is the youngest age a person has been known to have a face lift?

We had the experience of being consulted by the parents and their eighteen-year-old daughter concerning the necessities of a face lift to eliminate the ravages, scarring, and laxity of skin from acne. Dermatologists were unable to improve the general appearance of the facial skin by the use of their usual procedures—medications (ointments and lotions), dermal abrasion, or chemosurgery. The patient underwent dermal abrasion surgery with no apparent improvement. The young girl was despondent and introverted, and the parents sought help through plastic surgery.

A face lift on this young girl was deemed worth the trial to attempt to reduce the amount of sagging and reduce the depth of pitted scars by elevation of the muscles of the face and by putting slight tension on the skin. Excessive tension would be damaging to the muscle fibers; but mild stretch of the skin would be helpful. The surgery was sufficiently successful to restore the patient to normal activities. She is no longer a recluse.

Is there an ideal skin age or skin type for the face lift? What skin type is least responsive?

The ideal skin age for face lift, ironically, is the skin of youth—with only scant evidence of aging—a little wrinkling under the eyelid, a little deepening of the nasolabial groove, and only a slight amount of laxity of skin and fat under the chin.

The ideal skin is clear, pink, elastic, resilient, slightly plump, soft, and glistening with natural moisture. The common expression of "peaches and cream" complexion encompasses all these natural characteristics of a good skin. The skin is a good one when it has a healthy attractive glow without the benefit of cosmetics. We tend to forget the beauty of natural looking skin because our culture encourages the use of cosmetics from the adolescent years.

The earliest evidence of aging is the twenties when wrinkles begin to appear under the eyelids and at the outer canthus of the eyelids—first stage of "crow's feet." Therefore, the blepharoplasty is the surgery of choice for this young person.

The muscles of the face sag in the late thirties, and wrinkling becomes quite evident in the late forties. Men and women in their late forties and early fifties are in the ideal age group for face lift. This age group finds it most advantageous for physical improvement as well as social and economic advantage to resort to face lift surgery to restore youth. Fortunately, in most instances, people who entertain the idea of face lift surgery do appear at the surgeon's office at the correct age and correct time. The surgeon knows when he sees the patient in this age group that he has the best opportunity to restore youthful appearance. The reason is that there is still sufficient elasticity in the skin and the muscles of expression, which are elevated at the time of face lift.

Face lift performed on the patient in the late fifties and sixties provides great improvement, but the result will not last as long as the result obtained from the younger age group. The patient who has face lift in late years will return for a second face lift in a shorter span of time. This is understandable because of the natural and faster deterioration of the skin in this later age group.

The skin that is least responsive to successful face lift in the younger age group is the skin which has deteriorated because of physiological abuses: excessive drinking, smoking, eating, working, lack of sleep. Skin diseases such as acne destroy the quality of the skin. Excessive exposure to the ultraviolet rays of the sun and sun lamps destroys the skin. Poor quality cosmetics and excessive use of them are destructive of good skin. General physical condition as determined by the presence of debilitating diseases (cancer, tuberculosis, diabetes) is a factor in determining the quality of the skin. All or any of these factors which alter the quality of skin will decrease the expected surgical result of a face lift.

People beyond the age of seventy who show all the evidence of senility of the skin—yellowish or tan pallor, inelasticity, leathery texture, wrinkles, sags—is not ideal for face lift. The surgery will, however, reduce the amount of excess skin and in turn there will be fewer wrinkles and folds. The major area of improvement is the elimination of redundant facial skin and sagging of the neck. The elevation of the muscles and subcutaneous tissue and the elimination of the fat of the neck gives a firm foundation for the skin to be draped smoothly and sufficiently snug over the newly shaped chin and neckline. The elimination of the unattractive folds and wattles of the skin of the neck is most desired by the older age group seeking face lift. Ladies, in particular, want to be able to wear clothes that reveal a pleasing neckline. This is the feature that the older age group can improve with the face lift.

**Do you require payment in advance
for facial plastic surgery?**

The surgeon's office does not make a practice of establishing the credit reliability of his patients. His preoperative contact with the patient is often limited to one consultation visit. If the fee quoted is agreeable to the patient and the date of surgery is scheduled, the patient is usually requested to mail the fee to the office prior to hospital admission. An exception might be made for the patient who is a personal acquaintance of the surgeon.

**I have heard about silicone implants
and silicone injections. Can liquid
silicone be injected into the face to
eliminate wrinkles and face lines?**

Silicone implants can be used in solid form in facial plastic surgery for reconstruction and restoration of contour with anticipation of good results. The solid implants are used in the nose, the orbit, and the chin. Silicone implants are also used in the cheek to fill out deformities due to disease or injury.

Liquid silicone originally appeared to be a fine substance to inject into the skin as a filler for defects such as wrinkles and depressed scar areas. However, experimentation proved it unsatisfactory because the liquid silicone did not remain in the position in which it was placed by injection; it tended to stray from its site. Until the Federal Food and Drug Administration permits the use of liquid silicone for surgical purposes, the use of it should be avoided except under strictest experimental control.

**I have had liquid silicone injections
in my face. Can I still be considered
for face lift surgery?**

Although silicone injections for filling in facial lines and depressions are no longer acceptable surgical techniques, or at least performed only on an experimental basis at this time, their former application to a patient does not rule out face lift surgery. An inert substance, silicone has properties which render it harmless to the human body. Its tendency to stray from its intended position only means to the surgeon that the silicone material can be found in an unexpected or undesirable location when face lift surgery is being performed. If the surgeon does come upon a silicone deposit in the face, he can choose to try to remove it or ignore it, with the assumption that it would do no harm if it remains where found.

I take medication daily for an internal medical condition. Can I continue to take these pills while in the hospital for facial surgery?

A full disclosure of your medical problems is of critical importance in determining your suitability for surgery— any type of surgery. Since facial plastic surgery is most often elective, it would be foolhardy to submit to surgery of choice if you are not in good health. Facial plastic surgery does not encounter any of the vital internal body organs and, therefore, there is no danger in this regard; however, the drugs administered must not conflict with the drugs a patient is prescribed by a family physician or internist.

The ingestion of most drugs will not preclude a patient from undergoing facial plastic surgery. The medications can often be continued while you are in the hospital and recuperating postoperatively at home. Some drugs can frequently be halted for a few days before, during, and after facial surgery with no ill effects. However, cortisone drugs, medications for high blood pressure, and anticoagulants are of much more critical nature. The management of the drugs and the medical conditions they control make it absolutely essential that you discuss with your surgeon the medical problems involved.

In one type of facial plastic surgery, chemosurgery, the drug administered for deep chemical skin peeling is extremely harmful to the patient with kidney ailment. This patient would be told that chemosurgery is forbidden for him. It is advisable to hide nothing from the surgeon who wants to perform a successful operation.

How soon before a face lift may I have my hair bleached?

Hair bleaching and tinting may be done up to the day before you enter the hospital, provided that the process does not ordinarily leave your scalp irritated from the caustic elements in the chemical and bleaching agents.

Can a face lift be done under general anesthesia so that the patient is not awake?

General anesthesia is used by some surgeons, but it presents an additional hazard that need not be present in cosmetic face lift procedures. Most surgeons will discourage patients from this request because of the hazard of general anesthesia. Also, the muscle tone that is normally present disappears with general anesthesia so that the surgeon does not see your normal facial expression.

Cosmetic facial plastic surgery is performed well under local anesthesia. The surgeon can watch normal facial expression, even requesting that you smile, talk, or sit up, if necessary. The preoperative medications and injected anesthetic drugs are so effective that you feel absolutely no pain and will even enjoy cooperating with your surgeon to insure the best result possible.

What can I expect once I enter the operating room if I have only local anesthesia with face lift surgery?

In the operating room you will be received and transferred gently from a stretcher (actually a wheeled table) to the operating room table. You may even be asked to move yourself from the stretcher to the table, which you will be surprised to find yourself doing easily and eagerly. You will have had sufficient preoperative medication to feel confident, even euphoric, about your impending surgery.

Your surgeon may ask you to sit up in your room prior to surgery or when you are on the operating room table so that he can judge where you have the most sagging and wrinkling; when you are in a reclining position, many sags and wrinkles disappear or shift to another position. In the operating room the surgeon will review your photographs which were taken in his office at the time of your consultation visit or were taken by a professional photographer to whom he sent you. Evaluating what he sees in the photographs and how you appear to him at the time, he will finalize the details of your operation.

After completing surgery on one side of your face, the surgeon may request that you sit up once more so that he can determine the effect the surgery has had on your face. He sees then how you will look in several weeks, since at that moment you are not swollen as you will be in a few postoperative hours. Seeing you in the vertical position also enables him to decide how much tension to put on the other side of your face; it is not unusual to find more deformity on one side than the other. It also reassures the surgeon that none of your facial nerves have been affected or traumatized by the surgery.

During all this time, from the moment you entered the operating room, you are calm and complacent due to effective premedication at the bedside. If the surgeon notices that you are still slightly nervous or apprehensive he will not hesitate to order further medication, either more of the same you received preoperatively or an additional sedative or opiate like Valium or Demerol.

Rarely do we find a patient who is not completely at ease before the surgery commences. The patient who is not entirely at ease with all this medication might be administered a short-acting anesthetic such as Brevitol to get the procedure under way. For the rare patient who is completely uncontrollable, the surgeon will ask assistance. At that time a well-trained anesthesiologist enters the scene. He will administer anesthetics of only the safest type. You immediately go to sleep, are completely unaware of what is going on, and awaken in your room to find that your surgery has been completed. You are in good enough condition to eat the next meal served in the hospital!

How is the local anesthesia administered for the face lift operation?

Under sterile conditions the area that is to be the field of surgery is scrubbed with soap and water followed by an antiseptic. The surgeon, his assistant, and nurses are capped, masked, gowned, and gloved to guarantee sterility. Before any incisions are made, an abundant amount of a local anesthetic such as Xylocaine or Carbocaine with adrenalin is infiltrated under your skin. The surgeon chooses these anesthetics because they help control bleeding and are long lasting.

If the surgeon notices that you are having any discomfort from the operative procedure, he can immediately give you more of this local anesthetic. You are not expected to have any pain. The surgery should proceed smoothly for the good of all present. You, your surgeon, and the nurses are a team, and in order to have good teamwork everyone does his part to guarantee a successful conclusion to your operation.

How much hair is removed for a face lift operation?

About one inch of your hair is trimmed or shaved from behind the ear and into the scalp as far as the line of incision will extend. The surgeon is careful to remove no more hair than is necessary to provide him with a clear operating field. When the excess skin is removed and the incision is closed, the hair beyond the operative field is brought closer together and little of the trimmed area is exposed. The hair grows in the remaining trimmed area quickly in most patients. During the hair growth period,

the patient usually combs her own hair over this operated area.

On the male patient, sideburn hair is trimmed, as
well as a strip of hair in the temporal region and a strip
of hair behind the ear. Some of the sideburn growth
may be eliminated. However, the surgeon makes every
effort to give the patient a sideburn by rotating hair-
bearing skin of the face into the former sideburn area.

If hair-bearing skin needs to be placed behind the
ear in the rotation of the skin during the male face lift,
the surgeon may destroy the hair follicles before suturing the skin flap into place behind the ears.

**How much skin is removed in the face
lift operation?**

The amount of skin that is removed depends upon the
amount of excess skin present. If the skin is wrinkled
and atrophic in appearance, and if it has lost a great deal
of its elasticity, the surgeon may remove a greater
amount to attain the desired effect. It is borne in mind
at all times that when the wound edges are brought
together there must be no tension or pull on the skin
margins to be sutured together. Too much tension at
these margins will distort the angle of the mouth and ear
and produce scarring.

Elimination of facial sagging is obtained not by pulling skin but by elevating lax or sagging *muscles.* The
muscles of the face are drawn and anchored at their new
location by suturing. Good elevation of sagging muscles
can be obtained by the use of temporary plastic sutures
inserted into the muscles of the face and brought out on
the scalp. Two additional sutures of the nonabsorbable
type are placed on each side of the temporary sutures
and may be left there permanently. Temporary sutures
are removed about one week later. By this method of
face lift, more skin can be removed and less tension put
on the skin edges.

If a patient doesn't like hospitals,
can the face lift be done in the office?

Some plastic surgeons do face lift operations in the office. They may accommodate this request if they have an operating room within their office quarters similar to that of a hospital. There must be hospital equipment, instrumentation, and trained nursing assistance present. In most cases the operating room facilities in a surgeon's office are not adequate by normal operating room standards of the American Hospital Association. Good sterility is difficult to achieve in an office, as is well-trained nursing help. There is also the matter of insurance coverage, which usually reimburses a patient only when he is hospitalized for surgery.

Medical opinion is critical of surgery of the magnitude of a face lift being done in anything less than an officially approved hospital operating room. Emergencies can be treated rapidly and effectively in hospital facilities but may become a disaster in a surgeon's office. For these reasons fewer and fewer operative procedures are attempted in the surgeon's office.

Every precaution is taken to insure your safety and comfort in the well-managed hospitals of today. Moreover, your hospital stay is so short you will scarcely have time to decide whether or not you enjoyed it there.

When a face lift operation is performed,
is there a possibility of injuring a
facial nerve?

Yes, there is a possibility of injury to the facial nerves when a face lift is performed. Well aware of this danger, the surgeon brings his incision to the proper depth so as not to meet the facial nerves. He undermines the skin of the face at a specific level, leaving a little fat on the elevated skin.

The area in front of the ear is more prone to such an

accident, and here the surgeon uses the greatest care in undermining the skin. While he is operating, he watches for signs of twitching of the face, mouth, or eyes, which might indicate that he is approaching a branch of the facial nerve. Occasionally there is a facial nerve paralysis of the face immediately following the use of local anesthesia. This type of paralysis is temporary and disappears within several hours after the anesthesia wears off. If the facial nerve has been traumatized during surgery but not cut, paralysis may occur and last for several days.

If the facial nerve is severed the surgeon can immediately suture together the ends of the nerve. The patient's face will be paralyzed for several weeks until healing of the nerve is complete. The patient may also need physiotherapy to maintain muscle tone during the healing period. Fortunately, this surgical accident is practically unheard of today because of the excellent training of facial plastic surgeons.

A few of my friends have had face lift operations. On some I can see the scar line and on others I cannot see it. What mkes the difference?

The reason some scars are seen is that they are wide instead of fine hairline scars. Fine hairline scars are obtainable only when the surgeon can approximate the skin edges without any tension. He also avoids using any forceps to pull this tissue together so there will be no forceps marks on the skin. Numerous sutures have to be inserted with infinite care into a small area. Each suture has to be inserted at the correct level of the skin and through the entire thickness of the skin for the ultimate benefit of ideal tissue repair. Naturally, this is painstaking work and consumes an enormous amount of time. Your plastic surgeon will be prepared to take all this necessary time and effort to assure you as small a scar as possible.

Can I lose hair from a face lift operation?

Hair can be lost after face lift, but it is only temporary since the hair will grow back. The loss occurs because the normal blood supply to the scalp has been diminished, or the blood flow altered, due to the surgery. As soon as new blood vessels have formed and the temporary shock to the nerves of the scalp has disappeared, good hair growth will flourish again.

Permanent loss of hair is unusual. While you await regrowth of hair you can wear a wig.

What is a "mini" face lift? Is it cheaper than a full face lift?

The so-called "mini" face lift is really a partial face lift that is done either in front of the ear or behind the ear. "Mini" face lifts are an old story. They were practiced before the era of the total face lift as a cautious beginning by the early surgeons. The effects proved to be not only limited but insufficiently lasting to please the patient and the surgeon in proportion to the trouble and expense involved. Therefore, generally the plastic surgeon discourages such attempts except on the following occasions:

When the patient insists on a partial face lift despite the disadvantages cited by the surgeon; when by doing a partial face lift above the ear, the surgeon can reinstate a fallen eyebrow in a more normal position; when the relatively youthful patient wants early correction; when the patient has had a total face lift and wants only a limited correction a few years later; and when the perfectionist patient wants frequent but minor face lifts following a total face lift.

The fee for "mini" face lift is less than that of a total face lift and ranges from $500 to $1,000.

Will a face lift make the face look stiff or unnatural? Will a patient be able to smile normally?

A face lift is performed to eliminate sagging of the

muscles and excessive skin of the face and neck causing wrinkles and folds that are a sign of an aging face.

Smiling and other facial expressions are not altered. There is no stiffness or awkward feeling. Any pull and tautness of the face immediately after surgery are temporary and will disappear after several days. Normal postoperative swelling causes sensations of pulling and tightness of the skin. Some patients dread the gradual subsiding of this feeling, fearful that with the loss of tightness will go their new smooth look. To some small extent this happens. Normal resilience returns to the skin after swelling subsides, but usually just enough to bring back all natural facial movement and expression.

If a patient is satisfied with the way the skin of the face looks but notices the skin of the neck is too loose, can this be corrected?

Neck lift surgery is always performed simultaneously with total face lift surgery; rarely is it done as a separate procedure. The routine incisions around the ears and the undermining of the skin from behind the ears down to the neck prepare the way for lifting the excess of skin from the neck as well as the face.

After the final effects of the total face lift have been achieved, the surgeon readily realizes to what degree further elimination of the skin of the neck is necessary. This amount will not be as great as the one visualized before the face lift operation. The small correction needed can then be performed by making an incision under and behind the chin to remove the fat, to unite and reinforce the muscles underneath, and to excise the excess skin. This technique subscribed to and agreed upon by the patient after a clear explanation by the surgeon leaves the patient with a minimal scarring under the chin.

How many days must I plan to spend in the hospital when I have my face lift?

You must be prepared to spend three to four days in the hospital. You are admitted on the day before surgery in order to receive your preoperative diagnostic laboratory testing, a routine followed by hospitals and surgeons to protect you from undergoing surgery if you are not in normal health. The second day you have your operation. The following day or two postoperatively are spent in the hospital so that the surgeon may keep you under observation, change dressings when necessary, give you medications to keep you comfortable, and keep your spirits buoyed during the "blues" period immediately following surgery. The busy executive, male and female, often chooses to forego the comfort and convenience of an extra day or two in the hospital and arranges with the surgeon to be discharged as quickly as possible after the operation—sometimes on the day of surgery or the morning after surgery.

Is a face lift operation painful?

There is no reason for a patient to endure any pain from face lift surgery. Well-administered local anesthesia is effective in keeping you comfortable and free of any pain. Preoperative medication is started the night before your operation. In fact, you are frequently given medication as soon as you are admitted to the hospital to relax you and alleviate your normal feelings of fright and anxiety.

Most patients are so well medicated by the time surgery is begun that they are in light sleep, and although they respond if prompted by the surgeon, they rarely remember any details of the operation.

**May I wear my dentures in the hospital
and even during surgery? I dread being
seen without them.**

Your dentures are definitely to remain in place during and after surgery. It is desirable to maintain the normal contour of your mouth. Only when general anesthesia is to be used are the dentures removed before you are taken to the operating room. Even then, the surgeon may require that the dentures accompany you to the operating room so that he may decide if they should be inserted. If they are inserted, you are watched carefully by the anesthetist, who is alert to the fact that your dentures are in place during the time you are under anesthesia.

What is done following face lift surgery so that I am not frightened or in pain?

When you are brought back to your room following surgery, you are immediately made comfortable in bed. You may be frightened when you look at yourself in the mirror, and rightly so. If you have not been informed in advance that you will have a large dressing on your head and face, you might become alarmed. This large dressing is placed there for good reasons: to fix the tissues in place, to prevent bleeding under the tissues, and to minimize postoperative swelling. The dressing helps to immobilize the skin of your face just as a plaster cast is used to immobilize fractured bones. The dressing is bulky because the surgeon wishes to develop pressures at certain points. You may even find it difficult to speak with the dressing in place, but as soon as it is removed the usual motion in your lower jaw is restored. In most cases the large dressing is removed the morning following surgery.

You will have no pain following your operation. Your surgeon has written orders for you on your chart for medications to alleviate pain, and he is in constant touch with the nurses tending you concerning your condition and comfort.

What would I do if I have discomfort at home after face lift surgery?

To have discomfort after leaving the hospital is unusual for a patient who has had face lift surgery. If you do have pain or headache, you are advised not to take aspirin or Bufferin. You should call your surgeon, who will immediately prescribe for you such suitable medications as Darvon Plain or Tylenol with codeine, or any similar drug that does not contain aspirin. The reason for this is that studies have shown that aspirin can cause hemorrhage after surgery.

What bandages will I have on when I leave the hospital after my face lift surgery?

The large cocoonlike bandages placed around your face following surgery are removed the morning after surgery. The remaining small dressings which cover the sutures behind the ear and on the scalp will be removed on the fourth or fifth day postoperatively and replaced with new and still smaller dressings if needed. Since these dressings are inconspicuous they are easily covered by the patient's hair, a scarf or turban, or a wig. All dressings and most sutures are removed within seven days after surgery.

A few sutures are left in the face and scalp for about fourteen days. The hair of the head covers these, and they are not visible to anyone, including the patient.

How long must a patient stay home from work after a face lift operation?

Some patients leave the hospital the day after this operative procedure and return to their work a day or two later, if there is no unusual swelling or discoloration and the patient does not feel unduly weak. The female patient can cover her head dressings and sutures with her own hair, scarf, wig, or hairpiece and appear quite presentable. Men can also wear a hairpiece or use their own hair for coverage.

The usual postoperative patient can expect to return to work within one week with a wig covering any small dressings that might still be present. The use of wigs for men and women has been a boon for the person who must be on the go as quickly as possible after cosmetic facial surgery.

If there is swelling and discoloration as a side effect of the surgery, medication will hasten absorption of the subcutaneous fluids which cause the swelling.

I am told the face feels numb after face lift surgery. Is this true?

The feeling of numbness is a normal sequela of face lift. If it does occur, it may be the result of extensive undermining of the skin (separating the skin from the underlying subcutaneous tissues and muscles) necessary to eradicate all the excess skin and folds. In the process the surgeon will disturb some of the small nerve branches and nerve endings which carry the impulses of nerve sensation. The sensation of numbness can occur from the mere incision into the skin, which interrupts the nerve fibers. When complete postoperative healing takes place, normal sensation returns to the skin and this feeling of anesthesia, or numbness, disappears.

How long will a total face lift last?

A total face lift should last about five years. The quality of the skin, varying with each individual, is a determining factor. The skin with the heavier subcutaneous layer and more oil secretion from the dermal glands will maintain its firmness longer than the thin layered skin with its fine wrinkles. The thicker, oilier complexion ages with folds and sagging. The thinner skin ages with parchmentlike shallow creasing and fine wrinkles.

The male skin has a thicker epidermis reinforced by the hair follicles. The male face lift usually lasts longer than the female face lift because of this natural reinforcement. The mail hair follicles do for the male complexion what steel mesh does for concrete.

Fortunately, the face lift can be repeated successfully with little or no additional scarring, since the incisions in subsequent face lifts eliminate any visible scarring from the previous face lift.

What scars will show on the male face after the face lift?

No obvious scars will show following face lift surgery. One would have to look closely, perhaps with a magnifying glass, to see the healed scars. The slight redness of the scarred area, which is normal, disappears within several weeks. This redness is due to blood vessels that have grown into the scar area. It will disappear as healing takes place, since the blood vessels are squeezed in the web of fibrous tissue. As the fibrous tissue presses down on the blood vessels, the redness fades and the area is restored to the color of the remainder of the skin. Contemporary male hair styling provides excellent coverage for the fine incision lines that remain after face lift surgery. Hair pieces and false sideburns are also a great aid during the healing process.

If a man uses a makeup gel to look tan, can he continue to use this after a face lift?

The tanning makeup gels can be used readily. In fact they are a boon to the male whose face is exposed and unadorned without benefit of the female's source of beauty aids. The tanning gel gives the white man's skin a healthy appearance and tends to cover skin defects, including the faint scar lines of face lift surgery. The gel should be blended into the hairline, over and behind the ear (for incision line coverage) and onto the neck.

Is special makeup needed after a face lift?

Aging skin needs moisturizing. Cosmetic chemists have included a moisturizing agent in the formulary for most of the liquid-based makeup. It is easy to choose from the vast selection of cosmetic products with moisturizing agents one that will suit a patient as to color and smoothness of application. Powder should be used sparingly, if at all. The "shiny look" is considered young and clean, so a woman may refrain from the drying powders and matte finish makeups which tend to settle in the folds of the face.

The skin may be cleaned with water and a bland soap, glycerine, or one of the moisturizing makeup-removing liquid products manufactured specifically for the drying skin.

Overnight application of a thin, moisture-based liquid or cream that is absorbed by the skin, leaving just a faint film, is desirable.

Avoid makeup that emphasizes an antiseptic quality. The ingredients are not suitable for the aging skin.

Perfumes should not be applied to the skin, for they are drying due to the alcohol present in most perfume formulas.

"Toning" liquids in the cosmetic lines are pleasant and exhilarating but should be used sparingly. Most of these liquids have a witch hazel base and again encourage drying of the skin. If the toning agents are used to shrink puffiness around the eyes or the soft tissue areas of the face, they should be followed shortly by the moisturizer to counteract the drying quality.

Bear in mind that the youthful look is "clear of eye and pink of cheek." Your aim is to appear healthy, so use makeup sparingly and in flattering soft skin tones. Be sure to carry the color line over and onto the ears and down the neck (covering all incision marks).

Is it true that the sun is bad for the skin? After a face lift must I keep out of the sun?

The sun's ultraviolet rays are disastrously damaging to the human skin except in the mildest doses. The fairer the complexion the smaller the tolerable dosage. We cannot emphasize too strongly that the white male and female skin is unable to survive long the toasting it gets year after year by the sun worshipper, whether he or she is basking in the winter or summer sunshine.

Wind and frost add to the damages in ski season, and dry heat, plus ultraviolet rays, takes its toll in the summer season. Whether before or after face lift, the skin should never be baked, broiled, or sauteed in oil by the sun. Protective lotions and the largest brimmed hat that can be anchored on your head should be used when exposure is necessary. No one need miss a yacht trip in the Mediterranean as long as he or she is well shaded. The captain of the ship may look great with a tan, weather-beaten complexion, but you may hate yourself in a few years if your skin is equally creased and leathery.

Repeated overdoses of sunshine have sent many sun worshippers to the facial plastic surgeon hoping he can do surgical miracles so that the sun lovers can start from scratch. Normal skin aging does enough to destroy the plump smoothness of youthful complexions without exposing your face to the celestial fire.

If I don't like the result of a plastic surgeon's work, can I go to another plastic surgeon and expect him to do a correction or further face lift procedure?

If you are not satisfied with your appearance after a face lift operation, you should discuss your reasons with the operating surgeon. Did the surgery improve you but not fulfill all your expectations? Has anything happened to your face that caused an abnormality?

The feeling of dissatisfaction with the result of a face lift probably stems from the expectations you harbored prior to surgery. Your surgeon will explain what he did to improve your appearance within the limitations of your skin and the safe surgical procedures he must follow. How greatly you are improved in appearance may be less noticeable to you, who perhaps dreamed unrealistically of regaining a youthful complexion, than to others. Be truthful to yourself when you plan face lift surgery. There will be less chance of disappointment. Your plastic surgeon will explain what he can do for you. Listen carefully. If you do not understand fully how much correction is possible, ask for a clearer explanation of what you can anticipate.

When you are entirely aware of the degree of improvement that you have after your face lift surgery, and you still want another consultation, any plastic surgeon will discuss with you the possibility of further surgery. He will surely advise you to await complete healing before any decision is made. He may also want to talk with your operating surgeon.

In the rare instance when for some obvious reason the face lift is not entirely satisfactory, your operating surgeon will be the first to suggest and offer correction at the earliest opportunity.

Can a facial hair depilatory be used after a face lift operation?

If a facial depilatory has been used successfully and has caused no allergic reaction on the skin prior to face lift surgery, there is no contraindication for its use after surgery.

Face lift surgery does not change the chemistry or the texture of the skin. Where there were hair follicles that grew unwanted facial hair, the hair will continue to grow.

The elimination of this hair by use of a depilatory or by electrolysis is your decision. When excessive facial hair has been a serious problem, you should consult with a dermatologist as to the cause. He may find a medical cause or prescribe medication or suggest permanent hair removal, all of which can be safely done following face lift surgery.

**Can the habit of frowning bring the
return of deep frown lines after a
face lift?**

A frowning habit will have the same after effect on the
facial skin that it had before the face lift. It would,
therefore, be wise to try to overcome this facial habit.
Since frowning may stem from several correctable conditions, such as poor vision, photophobia, or living with
stress or tension, the patient should be checked by an
ophthalmologist and, perhaps, an internist or
psychiatrist.

**If a patient loses weight before the
face lift and then gains weight
following the operation, will this make
any difference in the surgical result?
What happens if a patient *loses*
weight after a face lift?**

The ideal time for a face lift is after weight loss, which
usually is accompanied by sagging of the facial skin. A
moderate gain in weight thereafter will not destroy the
effect of the surgery but will enhance the new, more
youthful appearance of the face. However, any further
uncontrolled gain in weight may unfavorably affect the
final result. To avoid this relapse, a patient should be in
the care of a physician interested in this special problem. He will make a study of an individual's nutrition
and advise accordingly. Weigh yourself regularly for
greater discipline. Remember you will have made a considerable investment in yourself with facial plastic surgery. This alone may deter you from transgression.

Many patients who have been ill and suffered severe
weight loss are startled to see what appears to be an
overnight aging. This is due to the loss of the fat layer of
the skin and the inability of the skin and muscles to be
"elastically" restored to their youthful firmness. With
health regained and weight restored, you will see im-

provement in the appearance of the skin, but seldom does the skin return to its former condition. Several years after your first face lift, and following a series of weight gains and losses that may have taken their toll on your face skin and muscles, you can have a second face lift.

How many times can a face lift be repeated?

A total face lift can be repeated several times and as often as necessary. Since a face lift operation has lasting effects for five to ten years, it is conceivable that the surgery, performed when you are about age forty, can be repeated every five to ten years thereafter, providing your general physical condition is good. "Mini" lift can be the recommendation for repeated face lift surgery on the patient who will not tolerate the appearance of aging skin.

I take sauna baths frequently. Will I be able to use sauna after face lift surgery? Is this type of dry heat beneficial or harmful to the facial skin?

You may continue taking sauna baths. With sauna the sweat glands of the skin are made to function at top efficiency, thereby ridding the skin of secretions and impurities that otherwise remain in the pores of the skin. The early period of dry heat does not adversely affect the skin like actinic (sun) rays. The dryness is quickly replaced by secretions and fluids (perspiration).

However, the beneficial effects of sauna are controversial. Some physicians feel the "baking" process is harmful to the complexion, which loses its natural moisture with aging. Excessive indulgence in sauna, like in other pleasures, can be harmful.

How soon after my face lift can I have my hair bleached?

You can have your hair bleached about four to six

weeks following your face lift surgery; by this time your sutures are removed, your incisions have healed, and your hair can be tinted with the necessary chemicals used in the dyeing process.

Shampooing hair can be done about one week following surgery, if you use a mild shampoo. No excessive rubbing of the scalp should be done at this time.

If you bleach your hair regularly, you should be reminded to have your hairdresser do the bleaching procedure about one week prior to surgery and then delay your postoperative bleaching as long as possible.

I wear a hearing aid. How long after face lift surgery can I wear my hearing aid?

You can wear your hearing aid three or four days after your face lift operation. If the hearing aid is the type worn behind the ear, you should delay its use several more days to avoid pressure on the suture lines. If your hearing aid is the type that fits into the ear canal, it may be worn as soon as swelling has subsided.

Will coworkers know that a person has had a face lift when the employee returns to work?

No. Others usually attribute your improved appearance to a new hair style, new makeup, fresh suntan (the new tanning gels do wonders for the male postoperative patient), gain or loss of a few pounds. In other words, almost any logical explanation is accepted by others for the improved appearance.

The scars need never give evidence of surgery, especially if they are healed well by the time the patient returns to the professional or social world.

Perhaps at some time in the future, when people accept plastic surgical correction as just another medical milestone, they will trade stories about their surgery and compare their incisions. A few public personalities have told their stories in print, thereby encouraging a more extroverted approach to this field of surgery. However, until the average person is willing to join this group of uninhibited and enlightened individuals, the world will not know who has had a face lift.

**What procedures must I follow to take
care of my skin after face lift?**

If we could halt our chronological aging, we would be taking care of our face lift in the best possible way. Since eternal youth is an interruption of aging not within our grasp, we must deal with the normal wear and tear of the years. To take care of our skin after face lift as well as our bodies, we must live a well-balanced lifestyle. Excesses of any kind cause aging. Normal physical and mental activities that stimulate the body and mind are healthful, and they are reflected in the condition of our skin.

In addition, cleaning the skin with mild soap and water, using moisturizer additives, and using protective sun-screening lotion against the sun's damaging rays all contribute to maintaining youthful skin after face lift surgery. Overuse of facial muscles in expressions should be avoided. Exposure to extreme cold and extreme heat is damaging to the skin. Temperate climate is kinder to the skin, and temperate climate with sufficient humidity is ideal. Tranquility of mind and absence of anxiety and worry prolong the results of a good face lift.

**Are retraining facial exercises
necessary after a face lift operation?**

Normal facial expression and muscle movement come naturally; no special facial muscle exercise is required after face lift surgery. As a matter of fact, manipulation of the skin by hand or mechanical massage should be avoided for three to six months following face lift. Only when there is an apparent paralysis of the muscles following surgery, a rare surgical complication, is it necessary to stimulate the muscles of the face.

**How long after a face lift can I again
use my razor?**

The steel blade safety razor can be used with a light hand several days after face lift. It can be used normally one week after surgery. The electric razor can be used earlier provided the patient moves the razor toward the scar line and does not apply pressure to areas of the face that appear discolored or swollen.

**I am a chain smoker. Can I smoke after
cosmetic facial surgery?**

No surgeon has forbidden a patient to smoke postoperatively if he has been returned safely to his hospital room and is fully recovered from the effects of anesthesia. Your surgeon may frown upon your addiction to smoking and personally disapprove of your anxious desire to smoke soon after surgery, but he will hardly choose that time to attempt to change your smoking habits.

**I had a face lift. Now I need to have
teeth removed and will require dentures.
Will this affect the result of my
face lift?**

Dentures are calculated to produce good occlusion and should maintain the ideal symmetry and harmony of your facial structures. The dental surgeon will reinsert your old dentures or new temporary dentures immediately after teeth extraction so that your face will not lose contour during your dental rehabilitation.

CONSULTATION WITH A PLASTIC SURGEON

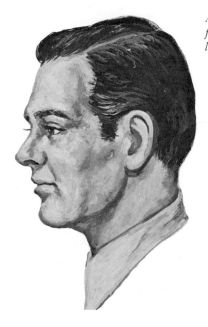

Age 40: Eye wrinkles and crow's feet; protrusion of eye fat; early laxity of skin.

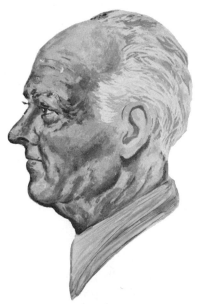

Age 60: Multiple folds of face due to loss of subcutaneous padding; loss of muscle tone; loss of elasticity of skin; prominent nasolabial fold.

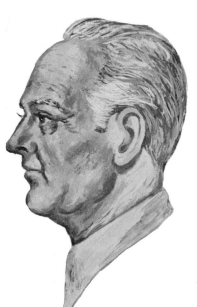

Age 50: Folds of skin around eyes; increased bagginess of lower lids; laxity of cheeks; chin sag.

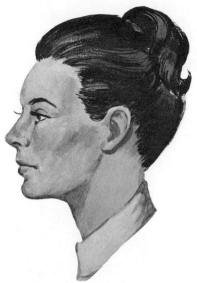

Age 35:
At age thirty-five you find the first appearance of some laxity and fleshiness under the chin. There is often the first sign of a mouth wrinkle and under eye sag. There may be some brow and eye wrinkle. The cheeks are usually smooth and well rounded; the nose and mouth areas are smooth.

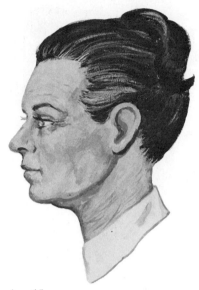

Age 45:
At age forty-five the pattern of crow's feet at the outer corner of the eye begins to emerge. The upper eyelid may have looser skin folds and the lower eyelids may have some protrusion of fat because of the laxity of tissues. The skin under the chin is looser and the mouth lines are more distinct.

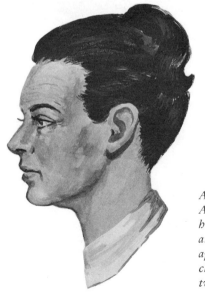

Age 40:
At age forty there are more forehead and eye wrinkles. The crease at the mouth—the nasolabial fold—appears more distinctly. Under the chin there is more laxity, and between the chin and the neck.

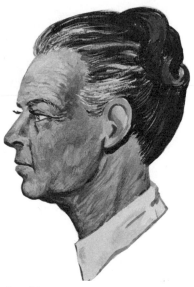

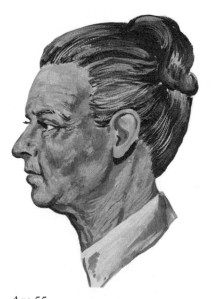

Age 50:
At age fifty the neck shows lines and more sagging under the chin. The cheeks are looser and begin to fall, forming the early jowls. The upper eyelids have more folds of skin and the out pouching is seen more distinctly in the lower eyelids. There are midforehead wrinkles and wrinkles at the root of the nose.

Age 55:
The laxity of the skin of the face at age fifty-five makes the cheek bones more prominent. The skin around the eyes has numerous folds and lines. The cheeks are loose and the skin gravitates downward, making creases around the ears, mouth, and jawline. The neck has vertical folds and deeper horizontal lines. There is considerably more laxity under the chin. In some people the cords of the neck will emerge distinctly; in others the flesh will form rolls of loose skin and fatty subcutaneous tissue.

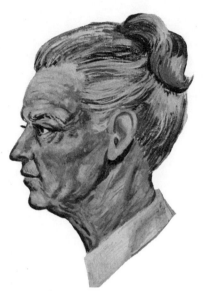

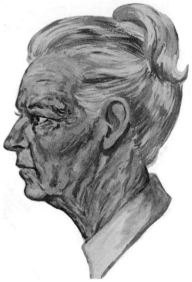

Age 60:

At age sixty the bony structure of the skull emerges more distinctly while the skin falls more as it loses the support of the muscles and the natural padding of the underlying tissue. The nose appears longer and the tip more drooping. The lower facial area appears slack and flaccid. The neck on some individuals can be extremely crepey with many creases and folds. The facial expression will reflect fatigue because of the pull downward of facial skin into the many vertical and oblique folds. The eyes are often quite heavy-lidded with a surplus of skin that sometimes droops below the margin of the upper eyelid.

Age 65:

At age sixty-five shrinkage of both bone and flesh takes place, and the head and face appear smaller. Folds and creases are deep around the mouth—from the nose to the mouth and from the mouth to the chin. The nasal tip is usually sharper and elongated. The neck skin is extremely loose and the neck has actually lost its contour. The skin from the face and neck seems to merge in common folds and deep creases. As a result there emerges the typical drooping "turkey gobbler's" formation under the chin with prominent vertical cords and sunken grooves between them.

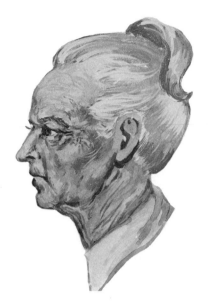

Age 70:
At age seventy the loose skin of the face usually has developed a network of small crisscross lines throughout, especially in the cheek area. This pattern of crosshatching gives the skin a leathery look. The nose becomes more prominent as the head appears smaller and bonier. The lip has many fine vertical lines and the mouth droops at the corners in the deep paralabial folds.

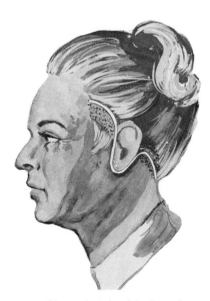

Excess skin undermined before elevation and excision. Incision line indicated.

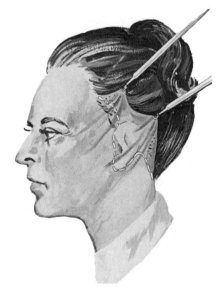

Excess skin elevated and excised in face lift procedure.

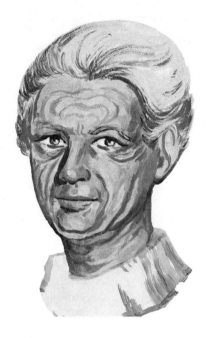

Facial Wrinkling: Nature's Design

Facial wrinkling is a natural facial characteristic, emerging at birth. All facial activity and expression cause facial wrinkling—smiling, crying, squinting, frowning, chewing, winking, talking. Every muscle in the face is prepared for action in many directions. The skin and its underlying tissues are like rubber, ready to bend and spring back in an instant. This wonderful face of ours is responsive to our every emotion, returning to its masklike smooth contour when we sleep.

However, although all function remains intact to old age, the face does not retain its beautiful contour and the skin does not retain its remarkable elasticity. The muscles become weak and overstretched. The fatty cushioning of the subcutaneous tissue gradually melts away. The skin, no longer supported firmly or cushioned plumply, droops and sags into folds and wrinkles as gravity drags it downward.

The wrinkle pattern which emerges with aging includes creases in all major directions: horizontal, oblique, and vertical. Horizontal grooves appear principally on the forehead and in the deep horizontal groove across the bridge of the nose. There are horizontal creases on the upper and lower eyelids and at the outer corners of the eyes. Oblique wrinkles, commonly known as crow's feet of the temples, soon fan out from the horizontal wrinkles. Vertical wrinkles occur in the furrows between eyebrows and on the upper lip, especially of women. A deep vertical wrinkling appears immediately in front of the ear. The most prominent oblique wrinkles appear from the nose to the angles of the mouth as an accentuation of the nasolabial fold and may extend further downward from the mouth to the chin.

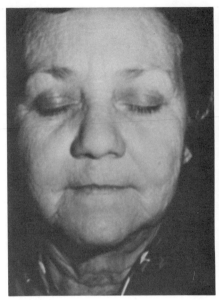
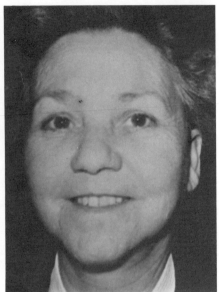

Face lift

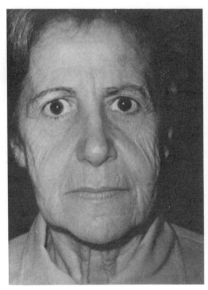
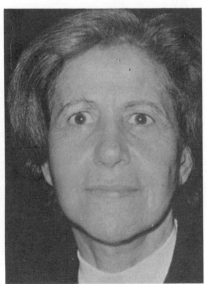

Face lift

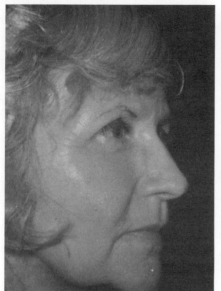
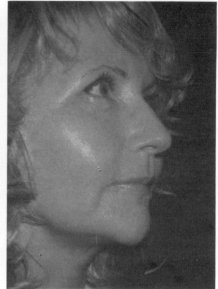

Face lift

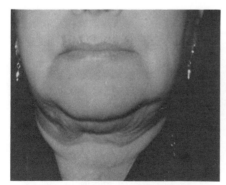
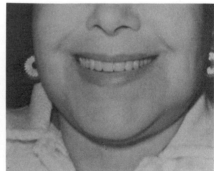

Neck lift

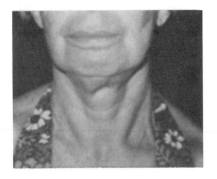
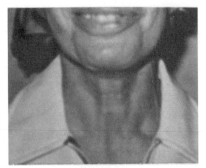

Neck lift

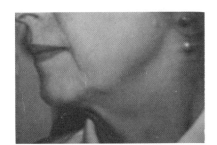
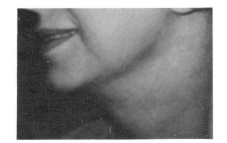

Neck lift

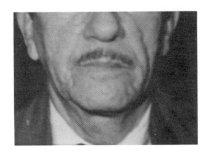
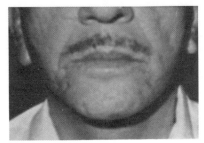

Neck lift

Face Lift for Bald-Headed Male
*Using horizontal incision from corner
of eye to ear.*

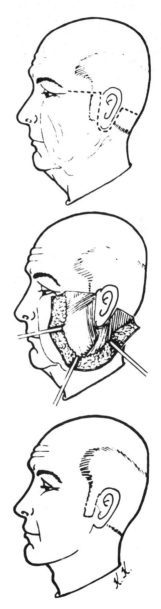

Operative procedure for male face lift

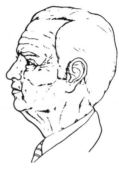

Loss of facial and eyelid skin elasticity and muscle tone in a male, age 65

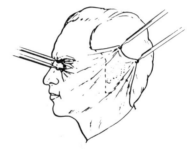

Removal of excess facial and eyelid skin and elevation of sagging muscles by corrective surgery

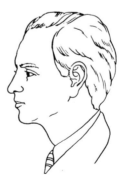

Ideal postoperative result following corrective facial and eyelid surgery

section 2

cosmetic nasal reconstruction

The disfigurement of a nose may be caused by an overgrowth or undergrowth in size, a congenital malformation due to an absence of some vital structural feature, or any distortion of shape out of the line of symmetry. Accidental injury can also cause disfigurement that destroys the beauty of the most prominent feature of the human face.

The prominence of the nose is accentuated by its being in view from five separate directions of eye gaze: head-on (front), right profile, left profile, from above (by the taller person looking down upon you), and from below (by the shorter person looking up at you).

The appearance of the nose is part of the whole scheme of the aesthetic quality of your face. As the three dimensional object between the eyes and the mouth, the two animated features that draw attention to the face, the nose is not meant to be poeticized or extolled for its own allure. If the nose interferes with the directional pattern of gaze, it is an obtrusion. Any deflection of person-to-person, eye-to-eye contact creates a serious barrier because the attention span is so brief. For two newly acquainted people to make contact a prompt responsive accord is required, and the fewer hurdles the better.

This does not mean that fame and fortune will elude the person with a deformed or unattractive nose. On the contrary, fame and fortune have come to some persons because of their nasal deformity, but only at the expense of their putting up with laughter and ridicule. Many great people have had "great noses," but they achieved success "despite" their nose. Psychologists will tell you many people succeed *because* they have a physical disability (cosmetic or functional); they are "overcoming" by "overcompensating." It is fine for those who have such stamina and who can disregard ridicule. We here are concerned for the average individual who desires to be accepted by society in all the usual areas of life, where appearance is one of the important values in interpersonal relationships.

The function of the nose is of critical importance in our analysis of the feature's place in facial plastic surgery. As the main entrance hall and corridor for the breath of life entering your body, the nose commands immediate attention if there is an obstruction.

All too often the person who has an unattractive external nose is also victimized by a deviated nasal corridor. This obstruction to breathing can be relieved and the cosmetic problem can be corrected at the same time. Here plastic surgery fulfills its dual purpose of restoring function and overcoming disfigurement.

The original surgical procedure for cosmetic nasal surgery was performed in Germany and Austria by rhinoplastic surgeons who used a small surgical saw that was placed under the skin of the nose to remove a hump from the nose. This method of rhinoplasty became the standard procedure for correcting the hump of the nose and refracturing the remaining nasal bones to narrow the nose. A refinement of the technique in present use by surgeons is an electrically powered saw, which saves a great deal of physical exertion. But most surgeons still follow the older and safer technique of the hand saw for reducing the size and the width of the nose.

Another technique developed for cosmetic rhinoplasty makes use of sharp edged chisels to cut away the nasal hump and to refracture the remaining nasal bones for narrowing the nose. The chisels vary in size to accommodate the variation of nasal shape and size. The advocates of this method stress that they can obtain a smooth, finely chiseled nose while avoiding the rough edges and the bone dust accumulating under the tissue from the sawing.

Well-trained, experienced rhinoplastic surgeons use one or both of these techniques today to correct the hooked, wide, or crooked nose. Both schools of surgeons use approximately the same method for shortening the nose and contouring the nasal tip.

The saddle nose (the nose that has a large depression of the bridge of the nose) is corrected by filling in the depression with cartilage, bone, or silicone. A good cosmetic result can be achieved by narrowing the nose and shortening and elevating the tip of the nose. This reconstruction can be performed at the same time if necessary.

The nose that is too short can be lengthened with the use of bone or silicone under the skin covering of the nose.

All these techniques for rhinoplasty, or nasal reconstruction, are performed instranasally (within the nose). Every attempt is made to avoid external scars. Reconstruction of wide nostrils are the exception to the rule because incisions must be made on the external nostril where it meets the fold of the cheek. Even in this approach a fine hairline scar results. Dark-skinned and black patients run a greater risk of discernible scars, and they are informed of this possibility prior to surgery. Also some black-skinned people are prone to keloids (large irregular scars). Ironically, most requests for narrowing of the characteristic flat, wide nose come from members of the race that must contend with the surgical risk of keloid scarring.

Regardless of the technique used, the surgeon's success in rhinoplasty is determined by the harmony of the facial features. And of course, the follies of Mother Nature are always with us. After a successful operation a patient may develop a nasal deformity unexpectedly because of the occasional fickleness of healing. This, however, is rather a rare happening.

Why is it that when I look at some people I know they have had cosmetic nose surgery? I don't want to have this telltale look.

Techniques of plastic surgery learned in the earlier stages of this field had certain telltale characteristics. One such technique caused the "pinched in" nostrils. The nose has a basically pleasant curvature and is well proportioned, but it is pulled in unnaturally at the tip of the nose. This results from removing skin with the lower lateral cartilages in the region of the nostril, the structure that determines the flare of the nostril.

Another technique which often has a telltale feature results in a roughly chiseled, as contrasted with a finely chiseled, nose. The front view of the nose is uneven, and the tip is likewise sharp and off center. The condition may be caused by the use of a surgical saw to hew down the bony support to achieve the curve. The saw, by its very nature of being an instrument that scrapes back and forth over the bone, creates rough edges. The saw also gives rise to bone dust and bone chips which are often impossible to eliminate entirely from the field of surgery. The result is a nose that looks uneven and whose rough edges can be felt by stroking the finger down the length of the nose, over the bridge, and over the tip.

Another "give away" feature is the scar or scars seen as a result of the early techniques of external incisions into the skin. The incisions left scars and made it evident that the person had had cosmetic nasal surgery.

The more modern techniques are a result of the vast improvement in rhinoplastic surgery. The more conservative handling of the lower lateral cartilages with no removal of skin and an intranasal approach result in a pleasing, normal looking nostril, with no external scarring. The use of chisels in place of saws results in the finely chiseled nose.

There is no reason for any patient today to appear to have had cosmetic nasal surgery. Although many patients are more than delighted to relate the story of their operations and to share the happiness of their new look, others are reluctant to reveal their surgical past.

I sleep with my mouth open. Can cosmetic nasal surgery change this?

Sleeping with one's mouth open is usually the result of a nasal obstruction due to a deviated septum, the central structure of the nose which separates the nose into two sides. A submucous resection is the surgery for correcting this type of nasal obstruction.

Cosmetic nasal surgery is usually done to improve the profile of the patient. Consequently this type of surgery would not be of benefit to the patient who sleeps with his mouth open. In some instances nasal obstruction is caused by an accident in which the bridge of the nose has been depressed or the nose has been pushed to the right or left. Cosmetic surgery will help in this case by improving the passage of air through the nasal airways and thus making mouth breathing unnecessary.

I snore in my sleep. Will cosmetic nasal surgery increase or decrease my snoring? Can I hope to eliminate snoring with nasal reconstruction?

Snoring in one's sleep is closely associated with mouth breathing. The person who snores usually sleeps with his mouth open. His whole respiratory system is gasping for air with each breath that he takes in his horizontal sleeping position.

The structures involved in snoring are an abnormally shaped soft palate, elongated uvula, and deviated septum. Snoring can be due to any or all of these conditions.

If the natural opening of the nose on one or both sides is obstructed by a deviated septum—curving off to the right or left—the flow of air is restricted. The obstruction may also be complicated by a swelling of the soft tissue lining of the nose due to allergies and upper respiratory infections (like the common cold). The air may not be able to enter the nasal passages as the sleeper struggles to breathe. As a result, he is usually snoring. Correcting the deviated septum by a submucous resection, and rhinoplasty if needed, will give the patient relief from his labored nasal respiration, thereby eliminating the snoring.

If the cause of the snoring is an elongated soft palate and pendulous uvula, snoring will not be eliminated by a rhinoplasty or a submucous resection. The offending uvula or soft palate must be shortened surgically. However, this procedure is highly controversial and has nothing to do with nasal plastic surgery.

Commonly, allergic children who experience blockage of the nasopharynx by swollen adenoids for a long period of time remain mouth breathers as adults. Many such persons must have orthodontia for malocclusion. Some patients are found to have a high-arched palate that shortens the vertical height of the septum between the floor and roof of the nose. The result is a restriction in the size of the nasal fossa and an inability to draw enough air through the nose to satisfy the requirements of normal breathing. They must open the mouth to breathe the supplementary air. They are lifetime mouth breathers. Until the orthodontist succeeds in achieving normal occlusion, a submucous resection or a rhinoplasty would not be helpful.

The tip of my nose droops. Can I have just this part of my nose corrected?

If only the tip of the nose droops and the remainder of the nose looks well proportioned to the face, the surgeon may agree that nasal tip surgery will give you a pleasing appearance. However, the plastic surgeon may not agree with your evaluation of the shape of your nose. It may be his opinion that only total cosmetic nasal surgey would give you the improvement you are obviously seeking. Bear in mind that each time plastic surgery is performed the final result must be as pleasing to the surgeon as it is to the patient. The plastic surgeon's reputation rides on your nose!

If surgery is performed only on the tip of the nose, no nasal fracture is required. The patient's face usually does not become discolored and swollen in the area of the eyelids, as with the total rhinoplasty. As a rule, the surgery is less traumatic and less costly to the patient.

However the surgeon should help you make the decision whether to have a total or partial rhinoplasty. A partial adjustment of the nose may not give you the harmonious result you are seeking.

I have chronic sinusitis. Can I have cosmetic nasal surgery?

Chronic sinusitis is not a contraindication to rhinoplasty. In fact, performed with a submucous resection and raising of the tip of the nose for the elongated nose the rhinoplasty may indeed improve nasal respiration by removing some of the obstacles to good nasal breathing.

However, chronic nasal sinusitis with swollen turbinates and nasal congestion and discharge is best dealt with by the surgeon as a separate surgical entity. Surgery on the sinuses may be carried out before or after the rhinoplasty.

When the sinusitis does not warrant surgery and is treatable medically, rhinoplasty can be performed without hesitation.

**What is the fee for cosmetic
nasal surgery?**

The average fee for rhinoplasty is $750. The range of charges by facial plastic surgeons throughout the country is $500 to $1,800.

**I don't like a pug nose or one not
suited to my face. Can you show me how
I would look with my new nose?**

Whenever a patient says he or she does not like a pug nose, we think of a pugilist who has taken too much punishment on the tip of his nose. Plastic surgeons have no objection to being told what you dislike. They will avoid giving you a pug nose, but please remember that they are well trained to give you the nose most suitable for your facial features.

Patients sometimes have set ideas about what their noses must look like. If their every request were honored by plastic surgeons, the results would be catastrophic.

If you are seeking the best cosmetic result in nasal surgery, permit the plastic surgeon free swinging of his scalpel. He needs latitude in his judgment and performance. If you allow him to use all his skill without any hindrances, you need have no fear.

At what age can I have a rhinoplasty?

Most facial plastic surgeons are of the opinion that age sixteen is an ideal age for cosmetic plastic surgery. The young adult is usually fully grown in facial features and height, although there could still be some growth period in the later teens, especially with boys. A fully grown fourteen- and fifteen-year-old can also be accepted as a patient for rhinoplasty. The surgeon will make his evaluation after he has examined the patient.

Because of functional problems reconstructive nasal surgery is sometimes required much earlier than this ideal age. Some children have so much nasal obstruction to breathing that to await the middle teens would be harmful to their growth, physical and psychological. Lack of air to the lungs through the nasal passages can stunt the development of the lungs and chest. Mouth breathing, which usually accompanies this problem, influences the development of the shape of the palate. The patient can develop facial features that are identified as the hawklike face of the mouth breather. Limited surgery of the nasal septum is indicated in these children to relieve obstruction to breathing, leaving the consideration of cosmetic appearance to a more appropriate age.

I am asthmatic. Can I have nasal plastic surgery?

There is no reason for an asthmatic or any other person afflicted with allergic conditions, such as hay fever, to avoid nasal surgery, provided the surgery is not done when the patient is in an active asthmatic or hay fever state. The patient should be properly treated for his allergies by an allergist or an otolaryngologist (ear, nose, and throat specialist).

Some asthmatics have an allergy based on an emotional involvement. These patients might be advised to have an examination by an internist and perhaps a psychiatrist. Emotional involvements can run the gamut from fear to sexual episodes. As one young female patient said to her plastic surgeon, "Doctor, please don't mistake my asthma for passion."

I suffer from hay fever. Can I have nasal plastic surgery?

Hay fever is a seasonal affliction, usually due to pollens of trees, grasses, and ragweed in your particular locale.

It occurs in early spring, summer, and fall. If you have been tested and found to be allergic to such pollens, you should have desensitizing injections to avoid seasonal discomfort.

If your condition is controlled during the hay fever seasons, there is no reason to avoid nasal surgery at any time of the year. If you have been treated merely with antihistamines for relief rather than desensitization, you are advised to avoid surgery during your hay fever season. If you are prone to sneezing during seasonal bouts of hay fever, your surgeon is able to control this situation with sufficient medications.

If I need a nose "lift," an eyelid correction, and a face lift, which should I choose first to make me look younger?

The degree of severity of all three conditions influences the decision in this dilemma. Also, the psychological trauma of the patient is of great consideration. Which of the three conditions does the patient dwell upon most often?

Let us consider cosmetic nasal surgery first. If the patient has a very elongated and/or a very bony prominence, this physical defect destroys the symmetry of the face which is the basis of our conception of beauty. Creating an appealing symmetrical nose may not assure a face to launch a thousand ships, but it is a positive step in the right direction.

Of particular value is the shortening of the drooping nasal'tip. Cosmetic nasal tip surgery can take ten years off the aging face. The uptilt of the nose is symbolic of youth. It evokes a definite reaction that causes us to use words such as "cute, adorable, sweet." The male whose drooping nasal tip is given a more straight chiseled appearance looks equally more youthful and more appealing in a masculine way.

The second choice in this conundrum of facial plas-

tic surgery is usually the eyelids. The viewer finds his
eyes drawn to the baggy eyelids on the face of the person at whom he is looking or with whom he is
conversing.

Therefore, according to the severity of either of the
conditions—the severely drooping nose or the baggy eyelids—the choice can be made. Both these corrections can
be made during the same operative procedure depending
upon the severity of the nasal deformity.

The face lift will also make the face appear younger
and, if all the other features of the face are symmetrical
and within the limits of attractiveness, the patient will
have enhanced his or her beauty.

Since the eyelid correction and face lift can be performed in one surgical procedure, this double-edged
scalpel technique will give the patient improvement in
two of three critical categories.

**Should I show the plastic surgeon a
photograph of someone whose nose shape
I would like to have?**

There is no objection to showing the plastic surgeon a
photograph of a nose you would like, but this does not
guarantee the result, for there are many factors that
influence the outcome, such as the shape of the nose
you start with, your particular features, your age, your
height, and nature's way of healing.

Your plastic surgeon will order photographs of you
on your first visit. You may be photographed in his
office, or you may be sent to a professional photographer. The surgeon may decide to show you a profile
of your future face by drawing some lines over your
photograph.

However, the surgeon can never promise you the
exact shape of nose he has outlined, but rest assured
that he will give you the most pleasing result possible.

**Some time ago I had a nasal fracture
in an accident. Now I want to have a**

**cosmetic nasal reconstruction. May I
claim I need this surgery to correct
the deformity which was a result of
the accidental injury?**

Nasal fracture due to accidental injury frequently causes nasal deformity. If the nasal bones were displaced, the reduction of the fracture may not result in the full restoration of the patient's former nasal shape. If the nose was of good symmetry before the fracture and is now deformed, this situation can be of grave consequence to the patient's peace of mind, and he is entitled to a cosmetic reconstruction of the nose after full healing of the fracture. In this case there is no question of the need for cosmetic nasal surgery.

If the patient's nose had obvious defects prior to fracture that are made worse by fracture, the opportunity for reconstruction is looked upon happily. The cosmetic surgery is still performed because of the offending nasal fracture, especially if the end result following the emergency treatment of the fracture was not satisfactory and provided the patient has waited six weeks to two months for complete healing of the fracture.

In the case of the patient who has had no change in appearance following the healing of a nasal fracture which caused no displacement (a fracture in place), cosmetic reconstruction is strictly a matter of choice. From this situation frequently arises a "sticky" question involving the legality of insurance claims. Many patients insist upon cosmetic nasal correction after fracture, claiming their noses do not look the same as they did previous to the fracture. Whether this is true or based on wishful thinking, the plastic surgeon who has not seen the patient before this fracture has no proof. Former photographs may be too indefinite to corroborate the patient's claim. The plastic surgeon, not wishing to place himself in judgment of the patient's credibility, accepts the history as told to him. For his records he may request a history of the case from the treating surgeon at the time of the fracture, or he may be interested in seeing the original X-rays, but he certainly does not do this to challenge the patient's description of his former appearance.

I would like my teenage child to have cosmetic nasal surgery, but he doesn't want it. Is there any way I can urge him to have this surgery?

This question is fraught with danger. The danger signs are twofold, "He doesn't want it," and "Is there any way I can urge him?" Cosmetic nasal surgery has no raison d'être if it is not a person's desire for improving his appearance. No one, male or female, young or old, should be dragged, coaxed, or bribed to see a plastic surgeon.

The psychological factor which plays so important a role in cosmetic surgery is a lethal weapon which can turn against the patient, his parent, and the cosmetic plastic surgeon. The young person who has no desire for plastic surgery can develop a self-consciousness about his appearance from the critical attitude of his well-meaning parent. His self-esteem can be damaged by his parent's lack of approval of his appearance. If he agrees to the surgery to please or quiet the critical parent, he will more likely reject his improved appearance than greet it happily.

The period of discomfort during and after surgery— short and mild as it is—will be magnified in intensity by the reluctant patient. He will more than likely be a headache to the surgeon and a heartache to his parents.

If the teenager has a gross physical nasal defect he may eventually request the needed surgery, because the mirror may speak "a thousand words," especially when he seeks out the mirror to see himself as some newly discovered romantic interest sees him. Here is where hope lies for his seeing himself as others see him.

If the nasal defect is a minor one, and only magnified by you as the well-meaning but misguided parent, your teenager will be satisfied with what he sees in the mirror and go on to his conquest with a confidence that should never be shaken.

Occasionally a youngster needs some encouragement to admit to himself that he needs and wants cosmetic nasal surgery. The suggestion and offer made by the parent to arrange and pay for the surgery are usually sufficient to arouse an interest in the teenager for cosmetic surgery, but the matter should be brought up only once and with some delicacy.

I know my teenager's nasal defect is a minor one, but he is very insistent upon having corrective nasal surgery. Do you approve?

Many people look at themselves more critically than necessary and develop an obsession about a mild defect. We tend to find these people neurotic, introverted, and extremely sensitive about their appearance. This hypersensitivity is particularly true of teenagers. Your youngster's minor defect may be of major importance to him and his self-esteem.

If the facial plastic surgeon sees the teenager's magnification of a minor nasal defect as indicative of some more major emotional problem, he will suggest that the young person be evaluated by a psychiatrist, who will determine the patient's suitability for surgery and share the responsibility of the decision with the surgeon.

Although nasal surgery is not always fully justified in terms of the degree of physical deformity, it may be completely justified for the mental health of the patient.

**I have a tendency to bleed profusely
when cut. Can I still have cosmetic
nasal surgery?**

If a patient has a tendency to excessive bleeding after injuries or minor lacerations or abrasions, he should give this information to the plastic surgeon at the first office visit. He will order additional blood tests in order to determine if there are elements absent in the blood that prevent normal clotting. Such abnormalities can be listed under the term "blood dyscrasia."

All patients receive a routine blood work-up when they are admitted to the hospital which would ordinarily reveal any abnormality. Should unexpected conditions develop when the surgery is actually under way, the surgeon can use special drugs at the operating table and surgical procedures to stop the bleeding.

If there is any reason to believe that the patient will bleed profusely because of nasal surgery, the plastic surgeon will refrain from operating. If there is only a possibility of profuse bleeding, the surgeon will have on hand in the operating room whole blood that is matched by type to the patient's. This precaution is rarely necessary as most patients are studied sufficiently well before surgery to insure safety.

**I have thick, oily skin. Can I
anticipate a good cosmetic result from
a rhinoplasty?**

A thick, oily skin does not necessarily present a problem to the rhinoplastic surgeon. The newly formed framework of the nose could be well covered by a substantially thick skin. Only occasionally will thick skin lack elasticity and not drape itself well over the new bony framework created by the surgeon. The result under these rare circumstances is less desirable, but there will still be correction of the deformed nose. The plastic surgeon will not be improving the quality of the skin with a rhinoplasty. Certainly he will not be able to change the thickness or control the oiliness of the skin of the nose.

How does one choose a surgeon to perform nasal plastic surgery?

Surgeons from two fields of specialty are uniquely trained to perform nasal plastic surgery: otolaryngologists, who specialize in facial plastic surgery, and general plastic surgeons. Consult your family physician for assistance in securing the names of surgeons qualified for this work in your community, or write to the specialty associations: the American Academy of Facial Plastic and Reconstructive Surgery or the American Society of Plastic Surgeons. The names and addresses of the current secretaries of these organizations may be obtained from your county medical society.

Can my Negroid shaped nose be changed to a Caucasian shape?

The Negroid nose can be reshaped to resemble a Caucasian nose by various interesting devices. The characteristics of the typical Negro nose are a flattening of the bridge of the nose, the tip, and the nostrils. The openings of the nostrils face straight ahead instead of downward as in the Caucasian. The nose is too wide for facial symmetry by some standards of beauty. Such a wide nose cannot be narrowed by the usual fracturing of the nasal bones. The narrowing can be achieved only by placing a silicone implant under the skin and over the bony skeleton of the nose. This projects the bridge of the nose.

The long and flat sides of the nostrils are shortened by removing a section from their juncture to the cheek at the nasolabial groove. The sides or wings of the nostrils can be rotated toward the midline and sewed in their new position. This rounds out the nostril, decreases its flatness, and raises the tip. If more projection is needed a flexible L-shaped silicone implant is used to project the bridge and tip at the same time.

By all these devices the plastic surgeon can arrive at a nose which tends to be more Caucasian and many times more functional for nasal breathing.

Complications may arise with surgery on persons with highly pigmented skin, such as the black race. They are prone to scarring and keloids (overgrowth of normal scar area). Since some of the incisions mentioned in the above technique are external and might give rise to keloids, the plastic surgeon will discuss this possibility with you and obtain your informed consent for this surgery.

Will I be asleep while I am having my rhinoplasty?

The anesthesia that is administered to rhinoplasty patients is the type that places the patient in a state of euphoria. Complete sleep is unnecessary because the surgeon knows the surgery can be done more safely if it is performed under local anesthesia.

General anesthesia is an additional hazard; moreover, the anesthetist is in the way of the surgeon. There is also much less bleeding with local anesthesia. As a result the operation can be done more rapidly and more accurately.

The ideal anesthesia consists of premedication the night before surgery and additional premedication before the patient is brought to the operating room. At the time of the operation, the nose is infiltrated with a local anesthetic, usually Xylocaine or Carbocaine, and no pain is felt thereafter.

Many patients fall asleep during surgery because they are so relaxed. If the surgeon wants to communicate with the patient during the operative procedure, he can easily arouse the patient from this light sleep.

At age fifty am I too old to have a total rhinoplasty? I have always wanted to have cosmetic nasal surgery but decided to wait until my children were grown. Will the nasal bones that need to be fractured for this procedure heal well at my age?

At age fifty you can unquestionably have cosmetic nasal surgery. This is not at all unusual. People have total nasal plastic surgery into their sixties.

The bones will heal well. However, the healing period may be a little longer than usual, but this should not deter the patient.

If the plastic surgeon is willing to do cosmetic nasal surgery on you at your age, he is confident that you will heal sufficiently well to obtain the cosmetic improvement that you are seeking.

I have seen people in the hospital after they have had a rhinoplasty. They have packing in their nose. This worries me. Will I be able to breathe with packings in my nose?

To breathe through your nose will be difficult for at least twenty-four hours after surgery. However, this should not disturb you, since mouth breathing automatically takes over and does an efficient job. Some surgeons insert tubes into the nose immediately after surgery and place packing around the tubes. The tubes are helpful in allowing some air to enter into the back of the nose and permit easy natural swallowing of foods and liquids.

On the second day, after the packing is removed, the patient feels a great sense of relief because the nasal passages are now adequate for good breathing. This, unfortunately, will be temporary, because within fifteen or twenty minutes nasal obstruction recurs due to the swelling of the intranasal soft tissues that follows the removal of nasal packings. Nose drops directed into the nasal passages every four hours alleviate the swelling and restore nasal breathing. Nasal drops are prescribed for the patient for the first several days following nasal surgery and are continued at home as long as the patient feels that the medication relieves the obstruction.

Other adjuncts like antihistamines and nose constricting agents taken by mouth aid in the reduction of swelling and improve the comfort of the patient during convalescence.

What is used to correct a depressed nose that has lost shape from past injury?

To improve the shape of a depressed nose following injury the surgeon will try first to use the tissues that are available in the nasal region. He will attempt to elevate the nasal bones if the injury is a recent one. If the injury is an old one, he still may be able to elevate the bones by loosening and resetting them.

If bone is missing because of absorption following injury or following infection resulting from injury, the nose may be elevated with the bone that remains. For example, if a nose still has a sufficient amount of nasal bones present and the nose is wide, the nasal bones that remain may be sufficient to eliminate the appearance of the depression. This procedure entails a nasal fracture which is performed by separating the nasal bones where they meet the cheek bones. The bones are then set in proper position and kept in place with an outer nasal dressing and internal nasal packing.

Where there are insufficient nasal bones to restore the natural contour of the nose, cartilage from the patient's septum or from the patient's ribs may be used. If the surgeon feels that cartilage is not suitable, bone from the crest of the pelvis (iliac crest bone graft) is available.

In the event that the patient objects to the use of bone from his pelvis, preserved human cartilage, which has been used extensively in the past for augmentation procedures of the nose, may be the surgeon's choice.

Today surgeons are making use of various synthetic materials, such as silicones. Methacrylates are now discarded because of tissue rejection and too great rigidity.

A great stride was made in plastic surgery when silicones became available. Liquid silicones injected into the nose for minor depressions tended to drift away from the injected area and were eventually discarded as unsuitable.

Solid silicones are today the ideal substances to use in the nose to correct bony depressions in the dorsum, inasmuch as the surgeon can easily carve a suitable graft at the operating table and insert it with little difficulty because of its flexibility. The use of this solid silicone makes it unnecessary to perform additional surgery to obtain donor cartilage or bone. The solid silicone, known as an inert substance, causes no tissue reaction. It does not change in shape or size as bone and cartilage do. Patients reexamined several years following solid silicone graft insertions show no loss of contour or absorption of the graft. The graft remained in good position and the skin is mobile over the graft. Silicone is most assuredly one of the miracle products of the last decade and has brought to cosmetic nasal surgery a safe and useful method for correcting the depressed nose. Although rejection of silicone as a foreign substance does occur, it is far less frequent than rejection of other materials used in plastic reconstructive surgery in the past.

**Will a rhinoplasty correct malfunctions
of the sense of smell or unpleasant
nasal speech?**

Malfunction of smell and nasal speech are most frequently caused by deviated septum, an internal nasal deformity which obstructs the normal passage of air through the nose into the pharynx, larynx, and lungs.

Any nasal obstruction to normal aeration of the nasal passages will disturb the normal sense of smell and the sound of speech. The external deformity of the nose is also partially responsible for disturbing speech and the sense of smell. A submucous resection to correct the deviation of the septum and a rhinoplasty to correct the external deformity are performed in combination for the greatest improvement of these two conditions.

Does the plastic surgeon take ethnic characteristics into consideration when building a new nose?

The patient who requests a rhinoplasty to correct a deformed nose is seeking the ideal aesthetic appearance of his nose and face. He wants features which are the accepted norms of beauty in our culture. The plastic surgeon is *not* concerned with the patient's ethnic background. He wants merely to perform a successful rhinoplasty by providing his patient with a well-shaped nose that functions well and conforms with his facial features.

Why is the summer a better time than the winter for nasal reconstruction?

Weather has no bearing on the rhinoplasty. In the past, physicians believed that because colds are more prevalent in the winter, nasal surgery should be postponed to the summer months. Air conditioning in homes and public places during summer months has become as much a source of chilling and colds as winter weather. However, it is important that the patient be free of signs and symptoms of a cold and upper respiratory infection at the time of surgery.

The physician instructs the patient following surgery to protect himself in winter or summer weather from upper respiratory infection by taking prescribed vitamins, particularly vitamin C, by dressing warmly when he is exposed to chilling air, and by not wetting his hair before exposure to cold.

All patients are instructed not to overexpose their faces to the sun during the first postoperative summer. That, of course, includes the patient who will visit tropical climates in the first winter following the operation. The patient must apply sun screening agents, such as Sol-Bar, Pre-Sun, or Coppertone, and wear visored hats for protection after surgery, if he is exposed to bright sunlight. Strong sun rays will burn the skin of the nose at a time when the blood supply has not returned completely to normal.

How long does the rhinoplasty take?
How many days will I be in the hospital?
How long must I be bandaged?

Rhinoplasty, or nasal reconstruction, takes about one hour of surgical time. The patient has an average hospital stay of three days. Nasal dressings held in place by adhesive tape are removed from the nose five or six days after the operation.

I understand that my nasal bones are
fractured during a rhinoplasty. This
sounds painful. How can I be sure I
will not feel any pain?

The local anesthesia used in rhinoplastic surgery is so effective, when administered by an experienced rhinoplastic surgeon, that you cannot feel any pain during any of the stages of the procedure, including the nasal fracture.

The premedications given the night before surgery and again approximately two hours before surgery makes you so comfortable that, by the time you are brought to the operating room, you are scarcely aware of the injections of painkilling drugs given by your surgeon as he prepares to operate. You will be only vaguely aware of your surroundings. You might even be in light sleep, as are most patients during their operation.

**Is it true that in middle age the nose
begins to droop and that a lift of the
nasal tip makes a person look younger?**

By the time a person reaches middle age—between forty and sixty years of age—the tip of the nose generally droops. This drooping is due to the normal relaxation of the skin of the nose which is, in turn, due to loss of elasticity of the skin.

The pull of gravity can also be blamed for drooping of the nasal tip. When the tissues no longer have the structural strength to withstand this drag, they fall earthward.

The surgical lift of the drooping nasal tip is simple for the cosmetic plastic surgeon to perform. It requires only an overnight hospitalization with a short recovery period. The patient can be back at his job in a week or less. Usually the eyes do not discolor nor is there any swelling of the face. The upper lip might feel taut and swollen but it does not appear so.

This procedure is a youth-restoring surgical technique because it changes the face in a most desirable fashion.

**If my nose looks too perfect after
corrective surgery, won't people know
that I have had plastic surgery?**

If it is a patient's desire to hide the fact that he or she has had cosmetic nasal surgery, the more perfect the nose the better the chances for dispelling the question of, "Did she or didn't she?" A nose that is apparently in good proportion to the face but has visible scars, rough bony prominences from spicules of bone, pinched in nostrils, and a pronounced curvature will more likely cause the viewer to wonder if plastic surgery has been performed.

A well-proportioned, softly curved (woman) or pleasingly straight (man), smooth-to-the touch nose will blend so well with the patient's facial features that a viewer would not think about the possibility of cosmetic nasal surgery having been done.

To the patient whose rhinoplasty is most successful but who still has not overcome the self-consciousness of looking pretty or handsome, we say, "Relax and enjoy it."

How long after my rhinoplasty can I engage in body contact sports?

The general opinion of plastic surgeons is that the nasal fracture done at the time of cosmetic nasal surgery takes about six weeks for complete healing. Although you appear quite presentable and can perform all duties and functions in about two or three weeks, you should not indulge in body contact sports for at least three months.

The danger of football, wrestling, and other vigorous contact sports is the risk of dislocation of the healing nasal bones fractured in rhinoplastic surgery. However, a deformity caused at this stage of healing can be repaired.

After the proper length of healing time has passed, the newly sculptured nose will withstand all the punishment that a normal nose could take. But just as it was a good idea to duck a severe blow to the nose with your old nose which didn't cost you anything, it is a good idea to duck with your new and more costly nose!

I have never had any trouble with breathing. Is there a possibility that a nasal correction for my deformity would cause obstruction to my breathing?

The chances are that if you have never had difficulty with breathing you will not have it following nasal surgery. The surgeon usually determines in his examination if you have normal or unusually narrow nasal passages, or a nasal obstruction due to a deviated septum. If you have either of these conditions, he will explain to you a procedure called a submucous resection that will help your breathing. This procedure can be done in addition to your cosmetic nasal surgery at the time of the operation. Cosmetic nasal surgery, however, should not cause difficulty with nasal breathing.

How can I be sure I will like my new nose? If I am not entire satisfied, can the plastic surgeon do a second operation?

There is no guarantee that you will like your new nose. However, every qualified and experienced plastic surgeon will naturally try to attain the best cosmetic result possible in your case. There is no reason why the surgeon should not take into account your wishes if they are reasonable and possible to carry out. But it is advantageous to allow the surgeon some freedom of action in achieving a nose that is most suitable for you. Knowledge of aesthetic values is part of his experience. The surgeon and patient should establish a common understanding.

Even after a skillfully performed operation, inevitably a period of healing ensues. Healing, as we all know, is not entirely within the control of the surgeon; it is something that partakes of the nature of the patient. Therefore, no surgeon can guarantee with absolute assurance a desired result.

Rarely is a result pleasing to the eyes of the surgeon but not fulfilling to the expectations of the patient. The surgeon has the option of not encouraging a second operation under these circumstances, especially if dissatisfaction with apparent improvement is combined with psychological disturbances.

In the instance where there is mutual agreement between patient and surgeon that a correction could bring further improvement, a secondary operative procedure can then be performed.

If I don't want to appear to have had nose surgery for cosmetic reasons, can

**I truthfully, or at least logically,
tell others that the surgeon changed
my nose because I could not breathe?**

It is entirely logical and quite often truthful that nose surgery is needed when there is an obstruction to nasal breathing. This can be due either to some deformity of the external nose or to a distortion or deviation of the nasal septum, which is the partition between the two sides of the nose. Both conditions may be present in the same nose. Nasal surgery is then indicated for their correction and to restore normal nasal breathing. The surgery would be both a submucous resection to correct the internal deformity and a rhinoplasty to correct the external deformity. The motivation for this surgery would be primarily for therapeutic purposes.

**How long after a rhinoplasty will my
face be discolored or "black
and blue"?**

Following a rhinoplasty your nose and eyelids will be swollen and your eyelids will be discolored. Sometimes the whites of the eyeballs (sclera) appear red because of blood that has escaped from the nasal area during or following surgery. This is called a subconjunctival hemorrhage and is nothing to be concerned about.

The swelling of the eyelids and the discoloration usually disappear within seven to ten days. Hemorrhage of the eyeballs also disappears in about ten days.

The nose appears swollen for about ten to fourteen days and this swelling is present when the dressing is removed.

The entire face can be swollen during this period as well. In some instances the area around the lower jaw and neck can show some discoloration, which is merely due to extravasation of blood to the lowest point. Blood weighs more than normal tissue fluids and tends to settle in the lower regions of the face.

Should I tell the person I marry that
I had my nose changed by surgery?

If a patient is seeking an answer based on the ethics involved in human relations, he might better ask a man of religion or a wise philosopher who can moralize on the subject of truth in marriage. If the question concerns the legal responsibilities of truth revelation at the time of marriage, a lawyer could draw on his judicial knowledge for an answer. If the question is based on the physical aspects of cosmetic nasal surgery, then the plastic surgeon can rightly give his opinion.

The facial plastic surgeon can assure you that there is nothing about a successful rhinoplasty that requires explanation or caution in physical activities. The newly married who has had cosmetic nasal surgery that is well healed need not fear injuring his nose in honeymoon tennis or sexual divertissement.

If the patient is plagued by feelings of guilt and equates having had cosmetic nasal surgery with something secretive about his earlier life, he should unburden himself at once by this innocuous revelation. Having had nasal surgery is no more revealing of one's vanity than using attractive makeup, having hair tinted, curled, or straightened, wearing a wig or hairpiece, dieting for slimness, or buying chic fashionable clothes. Being born to great beauty is so rare that one must face the fact that attempts at improvement are commonplace and of no earthshaking consequence to anyone.

Would having cosmetic nasal surgery
change my appearance to my young baby?
Could there be any disturbance in his
feelings toward his mother?

If the baby sees you shortly after your surgery has been performed, he may be slightly alarmed by your appearance, mainly because of the swelling and discoloration of the eyelids. But the baby will become accustomed to your new and changing appearance quickly and will accept the changes that he sees in your face daily. He will completely forget your former appearance. Even you and your friends will soon forget your former features. Patients have told their plastic surgeons that when they look over old photographs they are shocked to recall their former appearance.

When I make new acquaintances in the future after plastic surgery of the nose, will they know that I have had a nose job?

Cosmetic nasal surgery performed skillfully leaves no telltale evidence. Your nasal contour will blend with other facial features. In face-to-face encounters with new acquaintances the viewer reacts to a combination of factors—the smile that radiates the pleasure of a meeting, the warmth of your greeting, the directness of the eye-to-eye encounter, and the overall pleasantness of the facial appearance. Individual facial features, unless they are strikingly unattractive, will not command any viewer's attention. Self-consciousness about newly improved facial features should disappear in short order.

Would nasal surgery tend to change the hereditary characteristics in successive generations? If I have a rhinoplasty, will my children born subsequently have a nose similar to the one I had prior to surgery or after surgery?

Cosmetic nasal surgery does not alter hereditary characteristics in human beings. Genes which pass on inherited characteristics are not interrupted or distorted by any bodily surgery. Your children will carry the genes from both you and your mating partner. The features of your child can resemble your natural developed features, those of your mate, or a combination and refinement of both.

**Why is rhinoplasty called the most
unpredictable of operations?**

The many features and elements of nasal reconstruction
make its results unpredictable. The elevation of the skin
from its original framework interrupts the normal blood
supply; the remaining nasal bones and cartilage have
their blood supply altered when the nasal hump is removed and the bones are refractured; and the length of
the nose is altered when some cartilage is removed or
when the nose has its blood supply interfered with in
the reconstruction of the tip.

At the time of surgery or immediately afterward,
the soft tissue of the nose and eyelids swells and distorts
the appearance of the nose temporarily. Nature takes
over the healing of the reconstructed nose. New blood
supply to the skin must be redeveloped and the fractured bones must heal where the surgeon placed them.
Any variation of the normal pattern of healing can dis-
rupt the sequence of events of repair.

There can be collapse of the nasal framework due to
abnormal absorption or resettling of the nasal bones.
There can be temporary or permanent discoloration of
the skin due to poor blood supply. Blood elements can
seep under the skin or between layers of the skin, causing discoloration, temporary or permanent.

Some skin is so thin that blood elements remain
obvious and permanently discolor the skin of the lower
eyelids following nasal surgery. This explains the dark
rings under the eyes on patients who have had nasal
surgery.

The skin must readapt itself to its new framework.
Fortunately nature does its job well in most instances.
The elasticity of the skin permits it to redrape itself
around the new framework. This answers the popular
question of what happens to the excess skin when the
nose is made smaller.

Scar tissue is the end result of healing. This is nature's way of repairing tissues that have been severed and reattached to new positions. If nature does its job correctly (and fortunately it does with most people), very little scarring takes place during the healing phase, and a good cosmetic result is obtained. With some people, however, Mother Nature rebels, and she over-reacts with excessive formation of scar tissue, causing tissues to be pulled into abnormal position.

I wear eyeglasses all my waking hours. How soon after my nasal surgery can I wear my glasses?

You are reminded that you cannot use glasses that rest on the ears and nose too soon after a rhinoplasty be-cause a fracture of the nose has been performed to im-prove the nasal contour and the nose has an outside dressing for several days. As soon as the dressing is re-moved your glasses may be used, if they are not too heavy and if they are not worn for too long a period of time during the swollen, tender postoperative period.

Wearing any eyeglasses, especially those with heavy frames, too soon could impair the blood supply by the localized pressure on the healing nose. Patients seem to improvise the wearing of their glasses for seeing at a distance (the myope or nearsighted patient) or for reading (the presbyope or farsighted patient) by holding the glasses in a raised position over the nasal bridge and then removing them when the need ceases.

Ordinary spectacle wearing can be undertaken after ten days. In fact many patients wear colored lenses for a period postoperatively when the eyes are discolored or swollen from the surgery.

Where only nasal tip surgery has been done, glasses can be worn as soon as the outside dressing has been removed.

Contact lens wearers will be able to wear their lenses as soon as the swelling of the eyelids subsides.

**Can a person lose his sense of smell by
having a rhinoplasty?**

Rhinoplasty, or nasal reconstruction, merely changes
the shape of the nose. The olfactory nerve which sup-
plies the nose with the sense of smell is never involved in
a routine rhinoplasty procedure.

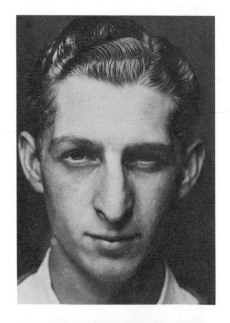

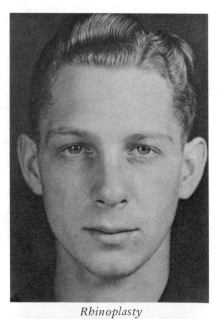

Rhinoplasty

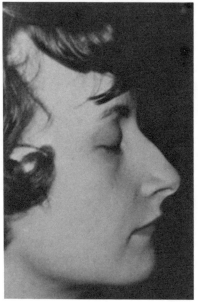

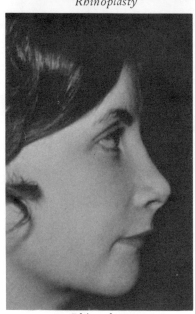

Rhinoplasty

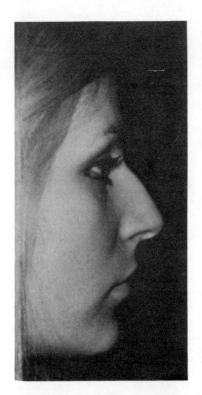

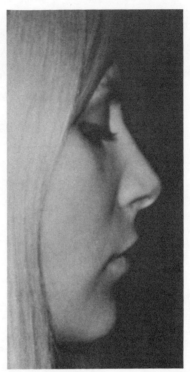

Rhinoplasty

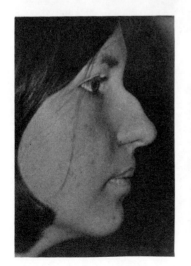

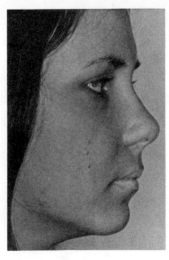

Rhinoplasty

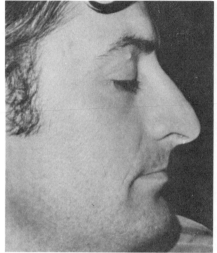
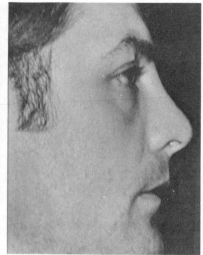

Rhinoplasty

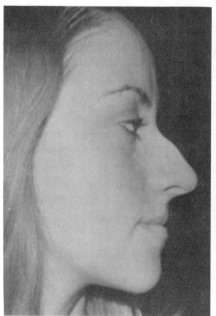
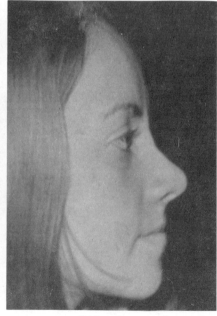

Rhinoplasty

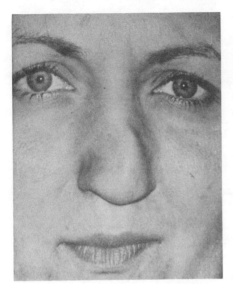
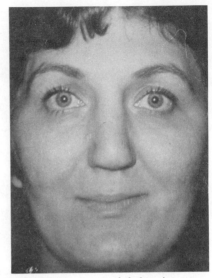

Rhinoplasty for nasal deformity

Corrective rhinoplasty

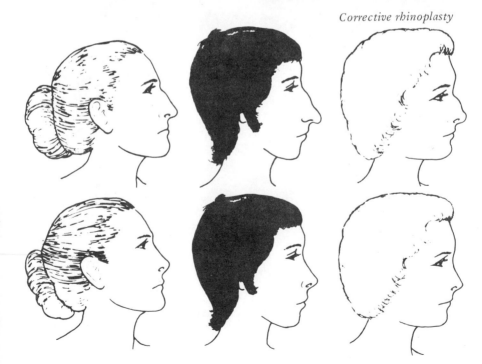

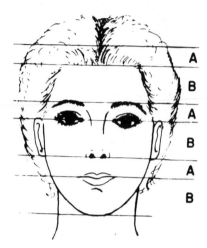

Ideal facial proportions:
Six divisions: A's alternating with
B's in a ratio of 1 to 2.

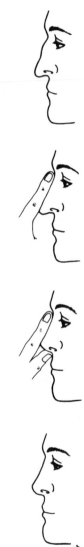

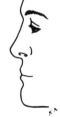

To estimate new nasal profile:
Eliminate hump with finger and
raise tip with thumb.

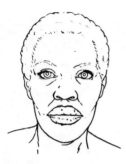

Preoperative:
Characteristic Negroid nose and lips

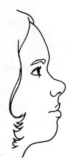

Preoperative: Depressed nose and
receding chin

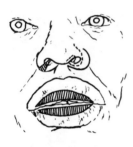

Operative procedure:
Striated areas to be excised in nose
and lips; rotated nostril as shown in
left ala.

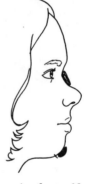

Silicone implants: Nose and chin

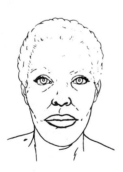

Postoperative:
Final result of corrective surgery.

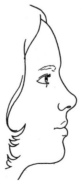

Postoperative: Silicone implants in
place

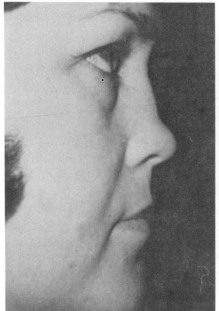
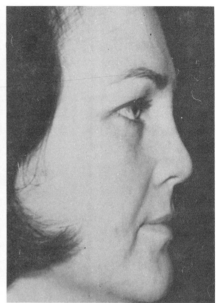

Rhinoplasty with silicone implant

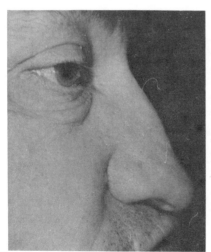
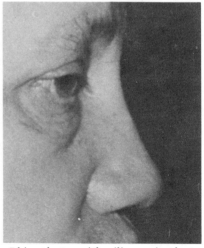

*Rhinoplasty with silicone implant
for deformed nose touching lip*

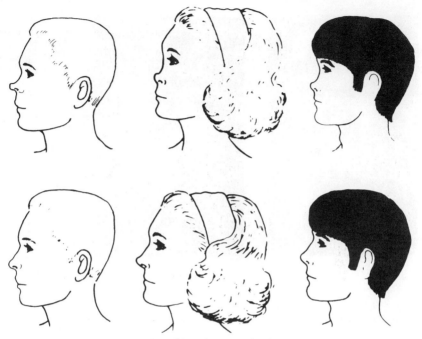

*Corrective rhinoplasty with silicone
implant*

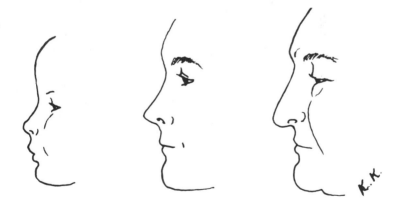

Influence of age on nasal profile

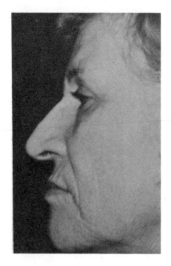 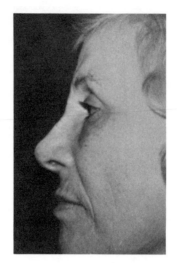

Rhinoplasty for more youthful appearance

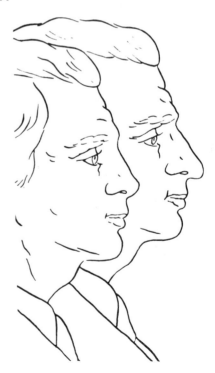

The nasal tilt of youth

section 3
cosmetic eyelid surgery

Your eyes tell the story of your life. The beholder of your eyes knows if you are happy or sad, calm or agitated, healthy or ill, rested or dissipated, young or old. The eyes with their window-drapery of eyelids must be sparkling, clear, and smooth-lidded to be the jewels in your face they are meant to be.

Mona Lisa's eyes have smiled upon the world for centuries, compelling us to look upon her beauty. Picasso, in his modern paintings, displays a grotesque but exciting emphasis of the eyes as the focal point of the human face.

We are, therefore, well-educated through our personal experiences and exposure to art and drama to look upon the eyes as vital to our general appearance. We want our eyes to reflect our beauty and strength. When they fall short of perfection we turn to improvement from outside sources—correction of vision by glasses or contact lenses, eye makeup for greater feminine allure, and cosmetic surgery for youth restoration.

Cosmetic eyelid surgery (blepharoplasty) is the most sought after surgery of the past-forty age group. The wrinkles, fat pads, and skin folds of the upper and lower eyelids give the first, most apparent signs of aging to an otherwise youthful face. We accept "laugh lines" rather good-humoredly, rationalizing this defect as giving the face "character," but the subsequent stages of skin degeneration around the eyes prove disconcerting and then unbearable to many middle-aged men and women. After trying astringents, creams, oils, vibrators, facial exercise, massage, eating and drinking more, eating and drinking less, vitamins, hormones, and "secret formulae" in dimly lit beauty salons, the frustrated victim of youth-restoration promoters finally turns to the plastic surgeon for help. Blepharoplasty is usually recommended and performed because it gives the relief the patient has been seeking.

The surgical repair of the aging eyelid is a painstaking procedure that requires skill, patience, and courage on the part of the patient and the surgeon. The structures involved are delicate and as exposed to public scrutiny as any anatomical structure can possibly be. Success is a necessity.

Beyond the cosmetic factor involved in blepharoplasty, there is the vital function of the eyelids to be accounted for. The eyelid, like a quick-drawing curtain, opens and closes to protect the eye against invading foreign particles, to circulate the tear layer over the cornea, to prevent drying by its blinking action, to shut out sudden blinding light, and to protect the eyeball during sleep. All these astounding functions are performed by the eyelids involuntarily because of the muscles and tissues present in the normal lid. Cosmetic eyelid surgery must remove the excess tissue and fat pads without disrupting the exquisitely precise actions of the eyelids. The trained facial plastic surgeon and ophthalmologist, aware of the limitations and danger areas in the blepharoplasty operation, avoids the over-correction of removing too much skin or damage to the muscles that control the actions of the lids. He follows the horizontal skin lines that nature provides to make scars almost imperceptible.

Blepharoplasty is performed for the less-than-perfectly-functioning eyelid. Here a reconstructive operation is designed to repair the results of the eccentricities of nature or the after-effects of accidental injury or surgery for malignancies. The plastic surgeon is then concerned with restoration of function first and cosmetic appearance second.

Cosmetic blepharoplasty has been performed more frequently on males within the last ten years. The great popularity of cosmetic blepharoplasty among females got its impetus with the use of glamorous eye cosmetics. These women who are eye conscious are now scrutinizing their husbands and urging them to rid themselves of their aging eyelids. It is not difficult to convince husbands and male friends that the results of this surgery are gratifying and certainly youth-restoring.

A group of people who require blepharoplasty are those whose aging eyelids take the form of a ptosis (falling downward) of the upper eyelid. The ptosis can be so extreme that the eyelids fall over the pupils of the eyes, causing an obstruction of vision. This drooping of the upper eyelids also causes a fanlike redundance of skin at the outer canthus (corner) of the upper eyelid which obstructs peripheral vision. Obstruction of vision can be further increased by the elevation of the lower eyelids because of a protuberance of fat (bagginess) which forces the lower lid upward. The combination of deformities causes a narrowing of the distance between upper and lower eyelids when the eye is open. The remaining space between the lids is called palpebral fissure. The smaller the palpebral fissure, the greater chance of obstruction to vision. Even when there is no obstruction to vision, the drooping eyelids and the small palpebral fissures give the patient a drowsy appearance. In some instances, the ptosis of the upper lids is so severe that the patient tilts his head backward to obtain unobstructed vision. Certain of these patients have an urgent need for blepharoplasty to correct the ptosis of the upper lids. The elevation of the lower lids caused by the fatty protuberance needs correction for the lower eyelid deformity as well.

Many elderly people have plaques of yellow infiltrated tissue consisting mainly of cholesterol deposits in and on the skin of the eyelids. These spots are called xanthelasmas. They appear in females more often than in males and are found mostly in the forties age group. These xanthelasmas can be removed at the time of cosmetic eyelid surgery. However, when they are numerous a combination of electrosurgery as well as excisional surgery must be used. Where the growths are excessively numerous, skin grafting is performed before the cosmetic eyelid surgery.

Wrinkles and fatty bulges of the eyelids can be congenital, appearing in the teens and early twenties. This deformity is no less a plague to the youthful adult than to the aging matron. There is no reason why the unhappy man or woman who has developed early signs of aging eyelids must accept this unattractive facial feature when surgical correction is possible. The technique used for the younger and older patient is essentially the same.

In the operative procedure the incision is made on the lower lid close to the border of the lid and in the upper lid in the fold of the lid. Anesthesia used is mainly local so that the patient, although sedated, can respond to any instruction by the surgeon to open or close the lids. The incisions extend slightly beyond the outer borders of the lid, curving downward for the lower lid and upward for the upper lid. This prevents distortion and allows the incision to fade into the natural lines of the eyelids. The amount of fatty tissue and skin removed depends upon the surgeon's judgment. In the younger person there may be no excess skin but merely excess fat to remove. The surgical technique used on the lower lid is more delicate and intricate than for the upper lid, so the major portion of operative time is spent on the lower lid correction.

Some surgeons use a dressing over the eyelids following surgery. The tendency is for the patient to reject this short period of blindfolding, and so most surgeons have abandoned this procedure of postoperative dressings. Merely covering the incisions with a medical eye ointment is sufficient.

The patient who has blepharoplasty will find this operation performed most frequently in a hospital and will have about a forty-eight hour stay. For the first few days following, the patient's eyelids may be slightly swollen and discolored, although some patients do not show any swelling or discoloration following surgery. Because the sutures are so small and are placed so close to the edge of the lower eyelids and in the fold of the upper eyelids, this patient can return to normal activity within a day or two after blepharoplasty. Surely the patient with excess skin and no protuberance of fat can be back at work almost immediately. Those patients who have some discoloration and swelling but feel otherwise ready to resume activity can use lightly tinted lenses or photogray sunglasses and resume normal indoor and outdoor activity.

Sutures are removed within four days of surgery. Early removal of the sutures prevents suture scars. If the surgeon prefers the sutures to remain in place longer, he will do what is called "subcuticular suturing." This suture material slides easily and removal is painless and leaves no marks.

Women patients should refrain from using eye cosmetics for at least ten days or two weeks to avoid infection and prolonged swelling because of the irritation produced by them. Since sutures are removed so early, patients are emphatically warned not to pull on the eyelids, for that could cause separation of skin edges.

Direct sunrays should also be avoided for several months after surgery.

Sagging, wrinkling, and superfluous skin are not expected to return for ten to fifteen years. The herniated fat forming baggy lower eyelids does not recur readily, even when the skin has a progressive degenerating tendency. The results of blepharoplasty are therefore gratifying to patients and plastic surgeons.

Certainly the patient needing both face lift and eyelid surgery who cannot afford or who cannot take the time off for both procedures at one time should have the eyelids corrected first. Youth restoration around the eyes offers great benefit to the aging face.

The aging face has its most dramatic rejuvenation in an operation which combines two aesthetic plastic surgical procedures—the blepharoplasty and the correction of the drooping nasal tip. More years can melt away in the simultaneous elimination of wrinkles and fat pads of the aging eyelids and the acquisition of a pert tilt of the nasal tip than in any other plastic surgical technique.

The blepharoplasty is a cosmetic surgical procedure that offers the most dramatic result for the patient and has the briefest period of recovery, but it requires the most painstaking skill of an aesthetic plastic surgeon.

I awaken most mornings with my eyelids swollen. This gradually subsides during the course of the day. Can I have cosmetic eyelid surgery despite this condition?

Morning eyelid swelling can be due to sinusitis, allergic conditions, kidney or thyroid disease. The cause in your case should be diagnosed by a history, physical examination, and any necessary laboratory and X-ray evaluation.

Puffiness will not disappear completely after eyelid surgery if you have sinus disease. You will first need conservative treatment with antibiotics, nasal medications, and possibly sinus irrigations to remove the source of infection and to help promote drainage of the sinuses. An otolaryngologist (ear, nose, and throat specialist) is the physician of choice for this treatment.

When the swelling of the lids is caused by allergies, the offending agent would have to be singled out by an allergist. You may need a series of injections to control the allergy.

If your swelling is due to a kidney or thyroid condition, your internist will probably do the required diagnostic laboratory and X-ray work-up to trace the cause of these ailments so that treatment can be planned for their control.

Where your eyelid swelling is marked, even though it occurs only in the morning, cosmetic eyelid surgery should be delayed until the cause is determined.

My upper eyelid makeup does not go on smoothly any longer. Can plastic surgery remove these extra folds of the upper eyelid?

Your aging eyelid acquires an accumulation of accordion-pleated loose skin that will not accept eyelid makeup attractively. Dry cosmetics cake in the eyelid folds and leave streaks. Cream cosmetics cannot be applied evenly for color or smoothness. The small protuberance of fat on the nasal side adds to the problem. The superfluous skin and fat should be removed to set the stage right again for the colorful scenery of eye makeup. The resulting scar is scarcely seen because it falls within the natural skin fold.

There are few complications to upper eyelid surgery. Occasionally too much skin may have been removed by the surgeon, but this incident happens so seldom that it creates no concern to experienced facial plastic surgeons, who can remedy the situation.

I have frequent excessive tearing of my eyes. Can I have cosmetic eyelid surgery?

Excessive tearing of the eyes is usually an indication of an infection in the tear ducts or tear sac. It can also be caused by inflammation of the lids or conjunctiva, allergies such as hay fever, corneal irritations, dusty environments, colds, glaucoma, and obstructions in the tear passages. Tearing is often stimulated or aggravated by wind or cold air. The lacrimal gland is producing an increase in the normal amount of tears passing through the usual tear passages and into the nose. When these passages are overburdened by the excess of tears, the overflow runs down the cheek.

Cosmetic eyelid surgery would not increase the severity of the tearing, but it would be neglectful of the plastic surgeon to proceed without advising you to consult an eye physician (ophthalmologist) for diagnosis and treatment.

Can I have my Oriental eyes "Westernized"?

Oriental eyes have been "Westernized" by skilled Japanese facial plastic surgeons for many years. American facial plastic surgeons have learned these techniques in the Orient and brought them back to our country to be used on individuals of Oriental-American origin seeking the Occidental look.

The so-called "epicanthus" is a congenital fold of skin between the upper and lower eyelids on the nasal side of the lids. This fold can be handled in a Z-plasty procedure which transfers the upper and lower flaps. The final scar is a faint one. Orientals, however, have a tendency to form keloids (overgrowth of skin). From the history and evidence of old scar healing, the surgeon can determine if this complication applies to you.

Another characteristic feature of the Oriental eye is a lack of horizontal skin fold in the upper eyelid and a protuberance of fat in the upper and lower eyelids. The absence of the skin fold is due to a short levator muscle (the muscle which elevates the eyelid) in the Oriental eyelid and to the muscle fiber structure (the end fibers do not reach the skin). In the Caucasian eyelid the muscle is longer and its fiber extensions enter the skin, thereby creating a fold in the upper eyelid. All that is required for the surgeon to create the fold is to bring the fibrous extensions of the muscle to the skin with several well-placed sutures, which are removed in about fourteen days. If the upper eyelid has excessive fat, an incision is made into the skin and the fat removed.

My lower eyelids turn out. Can this be corrected by plastic surgery?

An eversion of the eyelids, known as ectropion, is a condition of the lid where the margin turns outward and reveals the red or irritated conjunctival surface of the inner eyelid.

This condition occurs because of an injury or a relaxation of the lower lid tissues due to loss of muscle tone. A loose, flabby eyelid gradually elongates into a true deformity accompanied by annoying, unsightly tearing and irritation of the lid lining or conjunctiva. The condition can also be caused by paralysis of the orbicularis muscles or the surgeon's removing too much skin during a blepharoplasty for cosmetic surgery.

One of the methods of correcting ectropion is to shorten the elongated drooping lid by removing a section of tissue from the center of the lid and bringing the edges together. This should be done by an eye plastic surgeon.

The ectropion caused by a deficiency of eyelid skin can be corrected by a free graft performed by your plastic surgeon or eye plastic surgeon.

I have glaucoma. Is cosmetic eyelid surgery still possible for me?

Glaucoma, if well-controlled with the use of proper medication, should not in any way prevent you from having cosmetic eyelid surgery. Glaucoma is an intraocular disease caused by an increased pressure within the eye. The lid surgery is an extraocular procedure and does not affect or aggravate your glaucoma. However, you must tell your surgeon that you have glaucoma, and he will avoid the use of drugs that might increase the intraocular pressure. Your plastic surgeon will probably request clearance from your ophthalmologist to insure a safe and successful operation.

I have had cataracts removed. Is it
safe for me to have a blepharoplasty?

Cosmetic eyelid surgery can be performed on patients who have had unilateral or bilateral cataract extractions. The eyelid surgery in many instances improves vision as well as appearance. The excess of skin associated with senility of the upper eyelid can act as a curtain encroaching over the pupillary area if it falls below the eyelid margin.

The patient who is fitted with contact lenses following cataract extractions will certainly appreciate cosmetic eyelid surgery more than the patient who wears postoperative cataract glasses, since everyone is aware that these glasses are thick and tinted and actually mask the true appearance of the eyelids.

After your blepharoplasty, your plastic surgeon will require that you delay inserting contact lenses for about two weeks or until all signs of redness or inflammation have subsided.

My eyelids are darker than my facial
skin. Can something be done to lighten
the skin of my eyelids?

When the skin of the eyelids is of deeper pigmentation than the facial skin, chemosurgery is usually the suggested course of treatment, although results are not always entirely satisfactory. Acid application to the lids can create a depigmentation and therefore a lightening of the skin tone. However, it can also cause increased pigmentation, especially in people of dark complexion. If the skin of the eyelids appears dark and wrinkled as well, excision of the superfluous skin of the eyelids in itself will focus less attention on the darker pigmented eyelid skin.

Will I have both eyes bandaged if I have cosmetic eyelid surgery?

Some facial plastic surgeons do not place dressings on the eyes following cosmetic eyelid surgery. Other plastic surgeons prefer the application of eye dressings for a short time in order to reduce postoperative swelling and discoloration of the eyelids. When bleeding has not been completely controlled during the eyelid surgery and the surgeon is concerned with postoperative eyelid bleeding, he will apply dressings to prevent further bleeding. When so used, the dressing remains in place about twenty-four hours.

If you are to return to your room without an eye dressing, the surgeon may cover the incision lines with an antibiotic ointment. This alone in most instances is sufficient dressing for the incisions.

Bandaging both eyes is not the preferred method of most facial plastic surgeons because of the fright it induces in the patient, who returns from the operating room to find he must remain in total darkness with terrifying thoughts of having undergone surgery without knowing the result. Such a distressed patient could even convince himself that he has lost his eyesight. For psychological reasons elimination of the double eye dressing is desirable. The application of continuous iced compresses for a day or two is often used effectively by surgeons to control swelling and oozing of blood under the skin. Allowing you to see yourself in a mirror, even if you have sutures, ointment, and some swelling and discoloration, is reassuring that all has gone well. Plastic surgeons respect your fears and will not subject you to any unnecessary mental trauma.

My lower eyelids turn inward and the lashes scratch the cornea of my eyes. I

**have been advised to have surgery for
this condition. Can this surgery be
performed by a plastic surgeon?**

Your condition of the eyelid turning inward, entropion, is usually confined to the lower eyelids. This condition causes irritation of the cornea by the eyelashes. Correction of entropion is done by oculoplastic surgeons, who are ophthalmologists trained in reconstructive eyelid surgery. The operative technique results in a shortening of the lower eyelid and an eversion (turning out) of the eyelid margin and lashes.

**I have no loose skin under my eyes but
I have dark "rings" or "circles." I
always look tired. Can anything be done
for this?**

Your dark "circles" are visible when the veins under the thin and translucent skin of the lower lids are engorged. This in turn is due to congestion and swelling of the nasal tissues from rhinitis, sinusitis, or nasal allergy. The discoloration may be seen also in children. If the nasal congestion is relieved with treatment by an allergist or otolaryngologist, the darkness of the skin of the eyelids may disappear because the congestion in the nasal circulation has been relieved.

If the discoloration of the lids is due to hyperpigmentation because of increased melanin pigment granules in the skin of the lids, it may be removed by chemosurgery. This technique involves the careful applications of buffered phenol solution directly to the skin of the lids. While this treatment does not have an entirely predictable effect, in that the result may not match exactly the skin of the face, the new appearance is often a great improvement.

**My eyes protrude more than the average
person's. Will the scars of cosmetic
eyelid surgery be more noticeable on me?**

The scars will not be more evident because of protruding eyeballs (exophthalmos). The incision lines are made at the site of the normal fold of the upper eyelid and close to the lid margin of the lower eyelid.

Prominent eyeballs sometimes make deformities of the lids more noticeable. Removal of the skin and fat pouches under the lower eyelids and excessive skin folds of the upper lid will leave only an indiscernible fine hairline scar and will enhance the appearance of your eyes.

Can the fold of my upper eyelid, which is increasing in size and laxity, ever reach over the lid and obstruct my vision?

The folds of the upper eyelids will increase in number over the years sufficiently to fall over and below the lid margin in some individuals. If the folds fall two to three millimeters below the normal lid margin, they will encroach on the pupillary area of the eye, restricting the field of vision and preventing direct vision. The operative procedure for removing this redundant skin has been perfected and can be performed in the hospital, requiring of you a one- or two-day period of confinement.

I have fine crisscross lines on my lower eyelids that look like crocodile skin. Can plastic surgery correct this condition?

"Crocodile skin" appearance of the eyelids, a characteristic of the aging process in some people, can be corrected best by the use of chemosurgery.

Chemosurgery, a method of applying acids to the skin, will cause a second degree burn of the skin which will heal and leave a smooth layer of skin after the crust falls off.

True wrinkling of the skin with folds requires removal of the excess skin by surgery.

I have yellow raised patches on my
eyelid. Can they be removed?

> Your oval-shaped, yellow-orange patches raised above normal skin level (xanthelasma) can be removed by excision if they are small enough and do not result in too great a loss of skin tissue.

> If the xanthelasma to be removed are larger than can be excised and repaired in one surgical session, a series of operations can be planned for their gradual elimination to avoid loss of elasticity of the skin and prevent tension on the lids. If it is essential that as much be done as possible in one procedure, a skin graft can be used where there is available matching skin tissue from another lid.

> Electrocoagulation of xanthelasma is sometimes performed in suitable cases instead of excision, that is, if the areas of the skin involved are small and discrete.

If I do not want both my upper and lower
eyelids corrected in one procedure,
what would be the fee for separate
surgical procedures?

> The patient who has need for cosmetic eyelid surgery of only the upper or lower eyelids is usually quoted a slightly lower fee than a cosmetic eyelid procedure of upper and lower eyelids. If the surgeon's normal fee for eyelid surgery for four lids is $750, the fee for upper lids might be $350 and for lower lids $550-$600. If the surgeon's normal fee for corrective surgery of four eyelids is $1,500 (the upper limits), the fee for only upper or lower lids would be proportionately less.

What are the complications of cosmetic
eyelid surgery?

> Patients who undergo eyelid surgery can possibly have an eversion (turning out or pulling down) of the lower eyelid with the resulting tearing and exposure of the cornea of the eye when the patient tries to close his eyes (as in sleeping). This condition, if it occurs, can be cor-

rected by stretching and massaging the eyelid or by a surgical procedure which consists of taking superfluous skin from the upper eyelid and using it as a skin graft to the lower eyelid.

If too much skin is removed from the upper eyelid, the patient may experience difficulty when he attempts to close his eyes as in sleeping. However, this defect usually remedies itself several months following surgery.

Scars of upper and lower eyelids can be readily seen if the incision is made too low below the margin of the lower eyelid, or not close enough to the lid fold of the upper eyelid.

There can be an overgrowth of skin tissue during healing, causing a more obvious scar. For this reason surgeons are selective about the types of patients they choose for eyelid surgery. People with dark complexions (especially Orientals and blacks) are more prone to develop obvious scars.

The scars in some patients develop slight blisterlike formations where the sutures were inserted. These can be removed by your surgeon in the office. Blisterlike formations can also occur postoperatively on eyelid skin. These do eventually disappear.

Will cosmetic eyelid surgery, if not completely successful, ever interfere with vision?

Successful cosmetic eyelid surgery will more often *improve* vision than cause any loss of vision. In those cases that have a senile ptosis of the eyelids, surgery removes the obstruction to vision caused by the ptosis.

Cases of loss of vision following blepharoplasty have been reported in the medical literature. The explanation for these very rare occurrences is not entirely and scientifically classified at the present time. There may be well over several hundred thousand cases of blepharoplasty performed successfully yearly without any loss of vision. Only several cases out of the large number performed have been reported to have sustained loss of vision because of this operation.

One obvious reason for the loss of vision is uncontrollable hemorrhage in the orbit (eye socket), which can occur while the operation is going on or hours after the patient leaves the operating room. Another theory is an application of a too tight eye dressing, causing pressure on the eyeball and, in turn, on the optic nerve. Great pressure on the eyeball even for only ten or fifteen minutes can cut the blood supply to the optic nerve and eye, causing loss of vision.

As a safeguard, surgeons, at the time of the operation, clamp and tie blood vessels with suture material to obtain hemostasis (control of bleeding). Others will use electrocautery to obtain hemostasis instead of clamping and tying blood vessels. Investigators trying to determine the cause of visual loss in these rare cases have blamed the electrocautery technique as a possible source of trouble, citing that the electric current can go deeper than expected by the surgeon and can travel along blood vessels and nerve branches toward the optic nerve, which is located on the posterior wall of the eyeball.

Another complication of cosmetic eyelid surgery is the loss of the patient's ability to close the eyelid during sleep because of excision of too much skin of the eyelids, upper and lower or both. The cornea is exposed to the air and becomes dry and irritated. Only in the most extreme cases, however, would visual loss occur because of this complication.

The history of those few unfortunate cases of blindness recorded after a cosmetic blepharoplasty does not reveal the status of the eyes *before* surgery. It is impossible for those who are seeking scientific proof to judge whether it was or was not a previous condition that could account for the loss of vision.

What is the eyebrow lift that I have heard about?

As people age, the eyebrow, like other appendages of the body, droops from above to below the orbital ridge. This condition can be corrected directly, by excising an elliptical section of skin above the eyebrow, or indirectly, by removing an elliptical section of skin from behind the hairline and performing an upper face lift. Many surgeons prefer the indirect method because they hesitate to give the patient a scar near the border of the eyebrow. There is no doubt that this scar would be evident for many months following a direct eyebrow lift. The scar remains red until the blood vessels are obliterated by fibrous tissue formed during healing. The end result is usually a fine hairline scar.

Because of the inability to predict how nature will heal in certain areas of the body and especially because the eyebrow area is so prominent, many plastic surgeons are reluctant to perform this procedure unless they have specifically informed the patient of all possible complications.

Some young women seek an eyebrow lift to obtain an exotic appearance that comes from the upward sweep of the outer half of the eyebrow. This alluring characteristic gives the entire face a youthful elevation. When the falling eyebrow is lifted in the older age group, the upward sweep counteracts the appearance of the downward progression of the facial tissues caused by senility.

I am a photographic model in my early twenties, and I think that I have inherited eyebags. Can I have surgery to remove these so that they won't ruin my career?

This unfortunate development of eyebags at a youthful age can be corrected by the cosmetic surgical procedure of blepharoplasty. The procedure is performed by making an incision at the border of the lower eyelid and elevating the skin and muscle down to the bulging tissue. Here the surgeon finds fat and removes it. Although it appears as one mass, there may be three pockets of fat in the lower lid—one in the middle of the lower lid, another in the outer canthus, and a third in the region of the inner canthus. Only a small amount of fat need be removed to give a good cosmetic result. If too much fat is removed by the surgeon, an undesirable retraction of the lower lid results.

After the fat has been removed, the excess skin, if any, is trimmed and the skin edges are brought together with fine suturing. In most cases, no eye dressing is necessary. When the patient is returned to her room, cold compresses are applied directly to the eyelids to keep swelling and discoloration of the lids at a minimum. To prevent possible bleeding, patients are given vitamin K injections preoperatively and postoperatively. Infection in the region of the eyelids seldom occurs because of the ample blood supply to the lids.

Results of cosmetic eyelid surgery to remove eye-bags have been consistently excellent and predictable. The young woman whose career depends upon a youthful appearance as a photographic model will find that photographs will not reveal any evidence of her former bagginess following successful blepharoplasty, nor will the photographs show any evidence of scars from the surgery performed.

I have chronic edema around my eyes. Can plastic surgery permanently remove the puffiness?

The plastic surgeon makes a diagnosis first as to whether the puffiness is caused by edema (swelling) from a collection of fluid or whether it is a solid mass of tissue such as fat. If edema is the source of swelling, surgery is definitely not recommended. If the swelling is actually an accumulation of fat, surgery *is* recommended. The person who appears at a plastic surgeon's office for correction of edematous eyelids is frequently advised to

consult an internist to determine if the condition is associated with another medical problem, such as kidney or
thyroid disease.

**In an accidental injury I lost most of
my lower eyelashes. Is it possible to
restore them through surgery?**

Surgeons have constructed eyelashes for both the upper
and lower eyelids by excising hair with scalp from the
back of the head, making an incision near the lid margin
to insert therein this fine strip of scalp with hair. The
procedure is not entirely predictable for good and con-
sistent results. The insertion of a skin graft into the
eyelid may cause distortion due to scarring. The
changed direction of the hair growth toward the eyeball
can produce uncomfortable scratching of the eyeball.
The hairs may grow in a disorderly fashion so that constant care is needed to maintain the appearance of a
normal eyelash. It is preferable for the patient to
tolerate the application of false eyelashes to overcome
the deformity. False eyelashes are so well made, so
simple to apply, and can be trimmed so expertly by
cosmeticians to fit the eye that it seems foolhardy to
the average surgeon to attempt a delicate and dangerous
surgical operation when other means of cosmetic correction are readily available.

**My upper eyelids droop and look heavy
and tired in the evening after I have
done a day's work. Would cosmetic
eyelid surgery eliminate some of this
appearance of fatigue?**

The upper eyelids suffer an excess of skin in the older
ages. The weight of this excess must be lifted constantly
in normal winking and blinking. Blinking occurs every
four to five seconds. You can well imagine that by
evening this leads to considerable fatigue. You probably
find yourself unwilling or unable to read or to undertake writing tasks. Your evening out probably starts off

with someone commenting compassionately that you look very tired and must have had a hard day at the office. Actually fatigue has made your eyes look smaller and narrower. Your peripheral (side) vision may even be affected, causing some difficulty with night driving. An upper lid blepharoplasty would be extremely beneficial if you are bearing the burden of this excess skin and fat of the upper lids.

I wear contact lenses. How soon after eyelid surgery can I wear my contact lenses?

You can wear contact lenses about two weeks following cosmetic eyelid surgery provided there is no redness of the eyeballs or swelling of the lids. It is mainly the method of insertion and removal of contact lenses that makes it dangerous to use them before complete healing of the incision takes place. Pulling or stretching of the lids too soon after surgery may open the incision lines, necessitating reclosure of a gaping wound. The thin, sharp edges of the lenses can cause discomfort if there is still swelling and tenderness of the tissues.

Since you do not wear your contact lenses for several weeks after blepharoplasty, you should remember not to wear them for the usual full time on the first day of insertion, but to rebuild your tolerance for the lenses by a gradual daily increase in wearing time.

Can I lose my eyelashes with cosmetic eyelid surgery?

You will not lose your eyelashes when eyelid plastic surgery is properly done. Your plastic surgeon has been expertly trained in placement of incisions near the eyelashes. He always attempts to place the incision in a safe as well as inconspicuous area for upper and lower eyelids. The eyelid incisions are made some millimeters away from the edge of the lid and lash line to avoid injuring the roots of the lashes. It is uncommon for anyone to have eyelash loss following eyelid surgery.

**Will I be able to wear false eyelashes
after cosmetic eyelid surgery? The
adhesive used pulls the skin of the
eyelid when I remove the lashes.**

Do not use any false eyelashes or eye cosmetics after eyelid surgery until all redness of the eyeball has disappeared as well as the swelling of the lids. The nature of the adhesive used with false eyelashes does create a pulling action on the eyelid skin when the lashes are removed. When you resume wearing false eyelashes after the healing period, your eyelid will suffer no more damage from the pulling action than does the normal eyelid.

Between your wearings of false eyelashes, clean the thin liner surface of the lashes in order to minimize the amount of adhesive needed on the next wearing.

There are half-lashes that cover only the outer half of the lid margin above your own lashes, creating only one-half the pull necessary for removal.

Cosmeticians can apply individual lashes between and directly on your own lashes; these remain in place for several weeks. This technique eliminates the daily routine of applying and peeling off the false lashes.

**I wear eye makeup every day and feel
undressed without it. How long after
eyelid surgery can I use mascara
and eyeliner?**

The healing period after cosmetic eyelid surgery is usually about two weeks. The incision lines are close to the eyelashes and become inconspicuous shortly after the sutures are removed. After that, as soon as the redness of the eyeball and swelling of the lids have disappeared, you may safely wear your eye makeup.

**Is there any possibility of
visual disturbance after cosmetic
eyelid surgery?**

If too much excess skin in the upper eyelids is removed,

the patient is not able to close the eyes normally, leaving a gap that exposes the conjunctiva and cornea to drying because of insufficient wetting by the tears. The lids remain more separated during the night. Infections can complicate this drying of the exposed eyeball. All of this disturbs the vision because of the local irritation produced.

Fortunately, this entire sequence of unhappy events can be remedied by pulling the lids together before going to sleep and by inserting ointment into the eye at bedtime. Massage of the lids and the passage of time may shortly do away with this complication. If improvement does not result, then a free skin graft to the area of the eyelid where too much skin was removed will correct the condition.

If I have my eyelids corrected by plastic surgery, will the fit of my contact lenses be affected?

Following cosmetic eyelid surgery, your eyelids might be tighter than before and temporarily affect your usual contact lens wearing comfort. This discomfort usually disappears in several days since there are no noticeable changes in the shape of the cornea upon which your contact lens rests. If discomfort persists from contact lens wearing, by all means visit your ophthalmologist for a lens checkup.

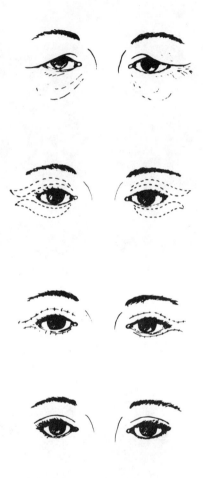

Blepharoplasty: removal of excess skin, crow's feet, and fat bags

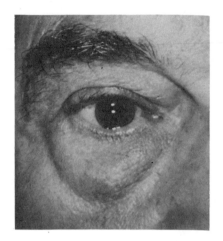 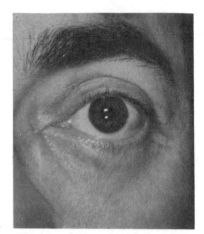

Blepharoplasty to remove excess skin and fat above and below eyes

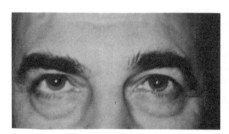 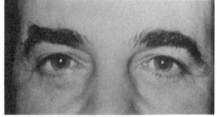

Blepharoplasty to remove pouches below eyes

section 4

dermal abrasion

Surgical skill and mechanical engineering are combined in the healing art of dermal abrasion. Nowhere is it more evident that a skilled hand must guide the machine, which is in this case a steel wire brush rotating at rapid speed. This immensely effective but lethal instrument is used by the trained facial plastic surgeon or dermatologist to remove scars, blemishes, and fine wrinkles of the face. Youth, the middle-aged, and the elderly benefit by this remarkable tool which cuts and scrapes the surface layers of the skin, eliminating defects in these layers. Nature performs its miracle, as it always does, allowing the skin to heal. The skin crusts on the surface while renewing itself below, and eventually the skin emerges as a fresh complexion. Not all defects of scarring and wrinkling can be eradicated, but improvement is heartily welcomed by the intelligent person who realizes there are no panaceas for severe deformities of the skin.

Dermal abrasion, an outgrowth of hand sandpaper abrading, depends upon the ability of the surgeon to anesthetize the face by quick freezing, to apply the sharp abrading wheel in the correct direction of the skin surface, to abrade and remove the scarred and wrinkled areas of the cheeks, nose, forehead, chin, and upper lip, and to accomplish this goal without causing postoperative scarring.

The surgeon will perform only what is safe and effective in his judgment with each surgical procedure. The patient will need only one dermal abrasion if his defects are minor, such as shallow wrinkles, freckles, hyperpigmentation, and acne, but he will need several abrasions if his defects are deep and extensive, as in deep-pitted scars of acne. The patient and surgeon are striving for the same degree of perfection—a complexion restored to a smooth, supple, healthy condition.

Because of the exposure of the face to the eyes of the world, there is a period of a few days in which the patient, having undergone dermal abrasion, will want to remain in privacy, since the postoperative state appears so distressing. The appearance, however, belies the true sensation, which is actually of little discomfort. After the scabs slough off, the patient feels free to be seen by the public, even if still "pink of cheek."

That the experience of dermal abrasion is truly not a traumatic one is borne out by the fact that it is often performed in the surgeon's office. The choice is usually that of the surgeon, who may prefer hospitalization for the patient.

Dermal abrasion is at this time being weighed against chemosurgery as to effectiveness for various types of skin defects. Surgeons who are trained well in one or the other method of treatment and have had successful results will tend to continue their usual modality. Surgeons who are trained in both methods of treatment will make a discriminating choice according to the condition presented for treatment.

The choice of whether to employ dermal abrasion for acne scarring, moles, hyperpigmentation, and fine wrinkling is as critical a part of the approach to this area of skin treatment as the treatment itself. There are sufficient variations in the skin from one individual to another as well as from one anatomical part to another on the same individual to warrant great care in diagnosis and choice of treatment. The regenerative powers of the skin are remarkable, and spectacular improvement is possible with dermal abrasion.

The fee range for dermal abrasion is $500 to $1,000.

How many dermal abrasion procedures will I need to eliminate my deep acne scars?

It is difficult, if not impossible, to appraise the amount of dermal abrasion that is necessary to eradicate deep scarring of acne. With many of the scars that are exceedingly deep their total depth cannot be reached by dermal abrasion. With each procedure there is further penetration of the pits and improvement of the appearance of the skin. The skin must be well healed before each successive dermal abrasion. The average patient who seeks this method of treatment for acne and pits due to acne seems to be satisfied after two dermal abrasions.

What is cryosurgery? Is it similar to dermal abrasion or chemosurgery?

Cryosurgery is a method of applying subzero liquid nitrogen to the skin by high pressure spray to "freeze" a blemish or lesion. The freezing of the blemish or lesion destroys the tissue, which will then slough off after crusting. What is actually happening to the tissue is similar to what a severe burn does to skin tissue. Cryosurgery is an "icy-cold" burn that penetrates the top layers of the skin in order to destroy an offending growth.

Cryosurgery, not at all a new technique to surgeons, is being used today to destroy acne blemishes, malignant skin lesions, birthmarks, warts, and many skin blemishes associated with aging skin.

The technique is extremely effective when handled with care by a competent specialist. Caution must be taken not to destroy healthy surrounding tissue, or to "freeze-burn" too deeply. To avoid scarring, the surgeon must not penetrate beyond the top layers of the skin. If you are familiar with the classifications of depths of burns, you will know there are first, second, and third degree burns. Cryosurgery attempts to effect a second degree burn, which will destroy the upper skin layer and cause a dried over crusting of the lesion, that sloughs off to leave a smooth, unblemished new skin.

The facial plastic surgeon or dermatologist will advise his patient if cryosurgery is suited to treat the acne condition or to attempt to remove the birthmarks or lesions involved. A frank discussion of the various techniques at hand for treatment and prospects of healing without scarring is in order in all skin problems.

I have heard of a technique for the improvement of the appearance of the skin called "dermaplaning." What is dermaplaning and how does it differ from dermal abrasion? Will dermaplaning remove my acne scars faster and more effectively than dermal abrasion?

Dermaplaning is a method of removing a layer of skin by the use of a mechanical skin planing machine. The removal of skin layers by the use of a sharp slicing machine has been an integral part of general plastic and reconstructive surgery for many years. Plastic surgeons have used a dermatome to remove a thin (or, at times, thick) layer of skin to transplant to a denuded area following serious burns or destructive loss of tissue from accidental injury or malignancy.

The use of a dermatome for "planing" the facial skin to eliminate scars or sick skin is limited by the permissible depth of dermaplaning to avoid scarring.

Dermaplaning is not synonymous with dermal abrasion, although the term is used loosely to imply a technique similar to dermabrading the skin. In one, dermal abrasion, the facial skin is mechanically abraded away (as is done by hand when one grates a potato). In the other technique, a layer of facial skin is mechanically removed in a thin slice.

There are surgeons who choose one technique over the other as most effective for removing the scars of skin disease. Most American surgeons choose dermal abrasion as more suitable for removing the top layer of skin of the face with minimum risk of permanent scarring.

I have been taking birth-control pills. After a vacation in the sun I found I had developed spots on my face and am now extremely sensitive to sunlight. Can these spots be removed by dermal abrasion? Can other medications also cause sensitivity to the sun's rays?

Your skin type is a determining factor in how sensitive you are to sunlight. The more melanin in your skin the greater protection you will have against the ultraviolet rays of the sun. However, there are drugs and chemicals that add to the vulnerability of a person to the damaging effects of the sun's rays. Among these are large doses of estrogen. Other medications that can add to light sensitivity are diuretics and even tranquilizers. Certain antibiotics could produce light sensitivity. Perfumes are offenders too. It might be a wise rule to follow to avoid sunbathing if you are on high dosages of any medication. Having incurred the blotchiness from exposure to the sun, you will probably have successful removal of these discolorations of the skin with dermal abrasion.

I have an acne condition. Will dermal abrasions help to eliminate active eruptions?

Let us make certain that you understand what has occurred in your body to cause acne. At the teenage growth period in your life, your body is producing hormones in an erratic fashion, which in turn is over-stimulating your oil glands. The oil glands thus stimulated begin to overproduce skin oil. Skin oil rises from its depression in the skin (follicle) to the surface, where it combines with skin debris and forms a thick white mixture (sebum). When the sebum reaches the skin surface and is exposed to the air, it becomes a blackhead because of a chemical change which takes place. Bacteria, always present on skin, will combine with the oil in the gland and cause an infection—a pimple or pustule. At this stage you are usually suffering externally (and emotionally) from your acne condition. How the pustules are resolved makes the difference between no residual scars or permanent pits of acne.

If the pustule ruptures spontaneously, it will leave no scar. But if it is harshly manipulated or is surgically relieved, scarring will occur. The infection often reaches the lower layers of the skin and causes permanent disfigurement.

Dermal abrasion has been successful in helping the acne patient in his active stage of acne and certainly in the stage of postacne scarring. Surgically abrading the top layers of the skin eliminates the pustule before it destroys the surrounding tissue (active stage) and reduces the depth of the scar pits already existing from previous eruptions.

**Is dermal abrasion the best way to
eliminate my acne scars?**

Dermal abrasion is the best known method for eliminating acne scars. By this method the top surface of the skin is removed where the acne is visible, and the scars of former eruption are penetrated with an instrumental procedure that smooths down the skin surface to reach near the bottom of the acne pits.

The procedure is relatively safe and painless when performed by experienced dermatologists or plastic surgeons. The healing is rapid and the results are gratifying.

Dermal abrasion can be performed by several

methods—mechanically by hand motion, using sand-paper, or by the more popular method, using a motor-driven, sterilized, wire brush which rotates rapidly. The patient's skin is frozen with a chemical to anesthetize the skin and to produce a firm skin surface for the moving and abrading wheel operated by the surgeon.

If your surgeon chooses to use general anesthesia, he may skip the freezing step and abrade directly on the skin. Healing will be the same.

More than one dermal abrasion may be needed to improve the skin sufficiently to satisfy you and your surgeon, particularly if the acne scars are deep.

Will dermal abrasion take away pouches and jowls?

Dermal abrasion is not suited to eradicate jowls, deep creases, or heavy wrinkling of the skin, but it is suitable for removing the faint crosshatch and shallow wrinkles of aging skin. Jowls of the lower jaw and neck and deep creases of the face are best handled surgically by the face lift procedure.

Jowls of the face and neck are the result of atrophy of the skin caused by senility. The condition is aggravated by gravity. The first sign of senility is a mere wrinkling of the skin. If this first stage of skin deformity is ignored and not corrected early by surgery, dermal abrasion, or chemosurgery, further advances of senility will aggravate the condition, causing redundant skin and jowls. This pathology of the skin is due to loss of elasticity in the elastic fibers of the skin and atrophy of the facial muscles.

When the facial muscles do not function correctly because of scarring of the muscle fibers, expressions such as smiling and laughing accentuate the appearance of the wrinkles, evidenced by the deep furrows and jowls. The jowls are accentuated further by loss of fat under the skin and loss of muscle tone. The skin sags because it is now too large for the framework of the facial bones. Only with the aid of facial plastic surgery, a face lift in this situation, can the tired muscles which have lost their muscle tone be elevated to their former location. The redundant skin is excised at the same time, leaving the face firm and smooth without pouches and jowls.

Should I have the warts on my face removed by dermal abrasion?

Warts are usually caused by a virus, and removal of warts by dermal abrasion is not scientifically sound. Warts can spread by manipulation of the viral tissue from one area to another. It is preferable to excise warts. Some small facial warts can be removed by electrocautery. Large warts will need surgical excision with extensive undermining of the skin flaps so that the skin edges can be brought together without any tension and can heal with a fine scar. When the wart is so large that the skin edges cannot be brought together without tension, the surgeon will use a skin graft.

When dermal abrasion is performed for removal of acne scars or fine wrinkles of the face, and there are warts or moles present on the skin, the surgeon will remove the blemishes surgically in his office several weeks in advance of the dermal abrasion.

Can the large tattoo on my arm be removed by dermal abrasion?

Dermal abrasion is most useful for improving the skin of the face. Attempts to apply the dermal abrasion method to skin of other areas on the body can be effective, but results are much less predictable.

The pigment used by the tattoo artist penetrates many of the skin layers. Dermal abrasion used safely will remove only part of the pigment, so that there will be a fading of the deep colors of the tattoo. Excision of the tattoo in stages until it is all removed is another more frequent plastic surgical procedure. Sections of the tattoo are removed surgically and the skin undermined and skin edges brought together. Several such operations will gradually eliminate a tattoo. A large tattoo on the body may even need a skin graft after excision.

I dislike my freckled face. Can the freckles be removed?

Freckles are superficial conglomerates of pigment in the skin produced by exposure to ultraviolet rays of the sun. They can be removed easily by dermal abrasion. Freckles on the body should not be removed by dermal abrasion because the skin on the body does not respond kindly to dermal abrasion. Scars may be the result of the poor healing following dermal abrasion of the body. Prominent freckles on the body can be eliminated with the careful application of trichlorocetic acid by a dermatologist or a plastic surgeon. Other methods of removing freckles are cryosurgery (freezing technique) and electrodissection.

During my pregnancy and even after giving birth I developed brown spots on my face. Should these be removed by dermal abrasion or chemosurgery?

You have developed a condition of the facial skin called "chloasma" or "mask of pregnancy"—brownish patches of pigmentation on the forehead, around the nose, and on the cheeks. This condition usually subsides after pregnancy is terminated with delivery. No surgical intervention is justifiable until sufficient time has passed to allow the hyperpigmentation to fade—about one year.

If you take birth-control pills, which are basically composed of female hormones and produce a condition similar to pregnancy, the hyperpigmentation may persist, increase, or return after its initial disappearance. When the pill is discontinued, the brown pigmented areas on the face fade or disappear.

As a woman with a tendency to this skin disturbance, you should be under the care and observation of a gynecologist, dermatologist, or plastic surgeon.

If the chloasma or hyperpigmentation of the face does not disappear with appropriate local and systemic medication, then dermal abrasion, which consists of surgical removal of the top layer of the skin, is found to be a successful treatment. Another successful treatment is chemosurgery, with the application of acids, such as phenol and trichloroacetic, to the face. This treatment, of course, should be done only by a physician trained in this procedure.

Can my skin tumor be removed by dermal abrasion instead of surgery, which would leave a scar?

No. If there is any doubt about your tumor, the surgeon will first request a biopsy. Tumors should be removed surgically and examined by a pathologist to determine whether they are benign or malignant. When the tumor is small, just removing a segment for biopsy is unwise; the tumor may be malignant and the malignant cells would spread. The careful surgeon will always try to remove any tumor by making incisions at a distance from the edge of the tumor. It is easy to understand that dermal abrasion, which destroys the tumor while scraping the skin, would destroy the evidence necessary for the pathologist to make an accurate diagnosis.

What is the difference in effect on my skin between dermal abrasion and chemosurgery?

In dermal abrasion, the outer layer of the skin is removed by a high speed wheel with a wire brush. The top layer of the skin is removed immediately. With chemosurgery the chemical cauterizes the skin and the cauterized tissue remains in place while new skin is formed beneath it.

Crusting of the top surface takes place in both instances. Immediate and thicker crusting starts several hours after dermal abrasion, whereas a thin surface of crusting starts two to three days following chemo-surgery.

In both cases the skin after peeling or crust removal is pink, tight as a drum, and smooth. Also, in both cases the exaggerated tightness subsides and the skin, although not as flawless as it appeared in the early stages, is nevertheless of a much finer texture and is relatively free of blemishes and wrinkles. The pinkness may remain for as long as twelve weeks.

If you are fair-skinned, either procedure will favor your result. If you are dark-skinned, you face more risk in the possibility of hyperpigmentation, which usually fades in a few months.

Both dermal abrasion and chemosurgery can be repeated several times without any harm to your skin since the skin restores itself to almost its original thickness. There must be a sufficient interval between treatments of an entire face, especially in chemosurgery because of the toxicity factor (for example, kidneys can be affected from the absorption of phenol).

Will the dermal abrasions change my skin so that I will not erupt with acne again in the future?

Following dermal abrasion to the skin for acne, the top layers of the skin with their accumulation of oil and debris in the skin follicles are abraded away, leaving a fresh skin layer without infected pustules. The disruption of the producing oil glands and elimination of the clogged pores are beneficial to the skin and will slow down if not eliminate further eruptions of fresh acne.

How long will I have to stay home after dermal abrasion? Can I have it done over a Christmas school holiday and appear normal when I go back to school?

Plan to be away from school for about ten to fourteen days after a dermal abrasion. Even after this period your skin will be bright pink for another few days. Cosmetics can be used to camouflage this rosiness of the skin without interfering with the normal healing process.

chemical skin peeling

Chemical skin peeling (chemosurgery) is an increasingly popular method for treating skin deformities by applying caustic chemicals to remove the outer layers of the skin (epidermis and upper layers of the dermis). The skin eventually sheds the "burned" layers to reveal a new skin which has formed beneath. This treatment is especially suitable for eliminating fine skin lines or shallow wrinkles, as around the lips, fine lines near the eyes (crow's feet), and fine creases in the cheek area.

Chemosurgery, also known as chemical peeling, is employed as one of the tools for rejuvenation of the aging face. The procedure sometimes follows a face lift operation when further refinement of the skin is desired.

Because of the many problems involved in handling unpredictable caustic chemicals on the skin, chemosurgery has not as yet been heartily embraced by all facial plastic surgeons or dermatologists.

A complete history, physical examination, and urinalysis should be required of every patient who desires chemosurgery to determine if there is any evidence of infection or damage to the kidneys. Because the basic ingredient of all chemical surgical formulas is phenol, which is known for its deleterious effect upon the kidneys, chemosurgery must be abandoned if the patient shows any evidence of abnormal kidney function or disease.

Chemosurgery involves too great a risk with certain qualities of skin. The skin which has had radiation treatment or shows evidence of having been burned usually lacks skin regenerating cells and will not heal well after chemical treatment. If the surgeon has a doubt about the skin's reaction to phenol, he may suggest a test be run. behind or in front of the ear near the hairline. If there is no evidence of scarring or discoloration after total healing of the test area, a full face chemical peel can be considered.

Phenol causes first and second degree burns of the skin with sloughing off of the upper layers. The burning action of the phenol is limited in its depth by the immediate coagulation process that takes place because of the combination of proteins and acid in the skin. The spontaneous coagulation process acts as a barrier to the deeper penetration of the acid into the skin and prevents third degree burns. If it were not for this immediate reaction and the protective quality of this protein-acid combination in the skin, the action of phenol would be entirely unpredictable and dangerous as a cosmetic agent.

After the acid has been applied with a cotton applicator or a brush, the skin blanches, and then several minutes later it becomes red and swollen. While the skin is undergoing a second degree burn, the patient feels the heat on the face for several minutes. The application of the chemical to the entire face takes about thirty minutes and is purposely performed in a slow, deliberate manner to reduce the speed and amount of absorption of the chemical through the skin. Too rapid and too great a quantity of phenol absorption by the blood stream could damage the kidneys. Kidney damage will result if the concentration of phenol in the blood is too high. If the fine kidney tissue is destroyed by high concentration of phenol before it can be eliminated, the mechanism of elimination of toxic elements from the blood stream will be upset. The patient will develop uremic poisoning.

Phenol formula application is usually confined to the skin of the face. If the neck requires treatment, the surgeon may continue painting this area slowly during another thirty minutes. The skin of the neck is delicate as it is thinner than the skin of the face and does not have the abundant blood supply nor the amount of subcutaneous tissue found on the face. Phenol formula must never be applied below the neck. When it is applied to the chest, scarring of the skin is almost certain.

During the period of redness and swelling, the skin secretes a clear fluid. The skin around the eyelids swells the eyes shut. After several hours the skin loses some of its redness and acquires a tan. Swelling persists for about four days but the painful period lasts for only the first several hours after application. Medication administered at this time will keep the patient comfortable. The swollen eyelids are treated with cold compresses.

After forty-eight hours the skin of the face begins to crust and the swelling begins to subside. As this process continues, by the fifth to seventh day, the crusts crack and crumble. As they loosen, the skin exudes serum from the crevices. After two weeks all crusting is gone, leaving the patient with a new layer of skin—pink, clear, and tight.

Following the initial application of phenol, the surgeon may increase the action of the chemical by allowing it to dry and then applying adhesive tape over the entire area treated. The adhesive dressing on the skin delays its normal stages of drying and scaling, thereby prolonging the period of action of the chemical and deepening its penetration of the skin layers. The surgeon's judgment of the quality of the patient's skin determines his decision to choose light treatment (chemical peel without adhesive dressing) or a deeper treatment (chemical peel with adhesive dressing).

The patient who is taped will have the tape removed in forty-eight hours. Since this process is painful, the surgeon may choose to use some sedation to keep the patient comfortable. A surgical powder which is dusted on the face forms a powder mask. One week later, and one day before this mask is washed away, the patient prepares the face with an application of a medical ointment or 'Crisco' to ease the separation of the powder mask from the skin of the face.

When the patient has undergone chemical surgery and looks at her smooth new skin with all crusts washed away, she is usually thrilled at the reflection she sees in the mirror. Unfortunately the appearance belies the fact that the tightness of her skin and the absence of the fine wrinkling is due partly to the swelling that is still present. The lines are "puffed out" by the unhealed skin tissue. As the swelling subsides some of the fine wrinkles and lines—linear and fine crosshatch—of the cheeks and lip area return, to the dismay of the patient! To allay this crushing disappointment the surgeon will forewarn the patient of this probability. The degree of expected improvement, even if less than hoped for, may be sufficient to keep the informed patient happy as the skin heals postoperatively. The fact that there are excellent temporary results and fair-to-good permanent results from chemosurgery encourages many women to go ahead with chemosurgical treatment; and the fact that chemical peeling can be repeated in certain limited, vulnerable areas (as around the lips) is comforting to the patient.

Patients who have dark complexions are forewarned that they run the risk of changes in skin color with chemosurgery. The skin may deepen in hue or form dark blotches. Usually this discoloration fades after several months, but it could last for several years.

Normal postoperative care following successful chemosurgery permits the use of soap and water after crusts are removed and a return to cosmetics about two weeks after initial phenol treatment. Exposure to the sun is forbidden for at least six months after chemosurgery because of the possibility of skin discoloration. The skin is highly sensitive to ultraviolet rays after chemical treatment. A good result from chemosurgery can keep the skin youthful looking for several years with good care by the patient who follows the advice of her surgeon.

Catastrophic chemical burns have occurred when this type of treatment has been performed by unqualified or inexperienced nonmedical personnel. Chemosurgery should be performed only by a dermatologist or a plastic surgeon who is well aware of the possible lethal effects of phenol. Complications of the skin treated with any of the phenol formulas or trichloroacetic acid or resorcinal can range from mild discoloration to grotesque and irreversible scarring of the skin of the face and neck.

Fees for chemosurgery range from $1,000 to $2,000.

Can chemosurgery of the face be performed on any patient or are there patients who cannot have chemosurgery?

Chemosurgery must be avoided by all patients who have diabetes, kidney disease, liver disease, heart disease, and a tendency to keloid formation. A person with poor nutritional status could suffer delay or complication in the healing process and should never undergo skin peeling with any type of chemical cauterant.

Chemosurgery is recommended only on the most ideal patient for this modality of facial plastic surgery—the fair-haired, fair-skinned, blue-eyed individual with fine wrinkles. If you fit these qualifications, you are likely to have the most success with chemosurgery.

I have heard that I can have face peeling, or chemosurgery, by a lay beautician instead of a medical doctor. Is that true?

Lay beauticians were the predominant group performing so-called "rejuvenation" for many years, and they have performed successful chemical cauterization on the face and neck. Unfortunately, their training and lack of scientific knowledge concerning the anatomical differences of the skin in various parts of the body and their tendency to disregard the toxic effects of absorbed phenol resulted in numerous cases of scarring and occasional death.

Even physicians cognizant of the above difficulties have at times still encountered problems with chemosurgery, and they have found the complications harrowing. The well-trained plastic surgeon must use all his skill and knowledge as a physician to minimize the hazards of chemosurgery. Therefore, it would seem the dangers encountered in this field should discourage you from engaging a lay person to undertake such a critical procedure.

Why are dark-complexioned people advised against chemosurgery?

Highly pigmented skin does not fare well with chemosurgery because of the dangers of hyperpigmentation following the application of caustics. Fortunately, the dark-complexioned person is less susceptible to early wrinkling and shows skin aging much later than fair-skinned individuals. The dark skin of the black race with its high melanin content has a natural protection against the ultraviolet assault of sunlight, and the elderly black person often appears deceptively young, even if he has worked many years in the sunny outdoors.

Hypertrophied scarring is common in the dark-complexioned patient. Attempts to eradicate the scar only bring another, and often larger, scar.

Would chemosurgery remove the deep skin lines on my face?

Chemosurgery is not at all suited to eliminate deep skin lines, but rather it is suited to eliminate *fine* wrinkling of the skin of the face. Eliminating deep folds of the face requires a face lift operation whereby the excess of skin is excised and suture reinforcement for the relaxed facial muscles is added. Chemical peeling is a topical treatment that is not meant to penetrate too deeply or to fill in deep crevices.

I have had previous chemical peeling and lost pigment on my face. Can this be corrected?

By injecting permanent pigment into the depigmented skin, the physician can blend it to your own complexion. This is actually a tattooing process. This technique requires a great deal of skill and acquaintance with the handling of the pigments involved. The mixture of the pigments and the injecting into the proper level of the skin are arts mastered by only a few plastic surgeons and technicians. This process is slow, laborious, time-consuming, and costly.

This same process can be used in reverse to take out color or to lighten deeply colored blemishes like port wine stains (birthmarks).

I am interested in having chemical peeling and have studied some chemistry. Do I have a choice of acids? What would be those from which I could choose?

There are several chemicals that are used by facial plastic surgeons and dermatologists to attempt to achieve the new unwrinkled or unblemished skin you are seeking. They are of varying degrees of effectiveness according to their penetration of the skin layers, their method of application, and their properties for permitting the skin to heal with the least amount of damage.

These chemicals are resorcinol, lactic acid, benzoic acid, salicylic acid, trichloroacetic acid, and phenol. The first four chemicals are called superficial exfoliants by the profession since they do not produce the deep beneficial effects.

Trichloroacetic acid is effective but so powerful a corrosive that it can cause much deeper destruction than desired. Because of this property, trichloroacetic acid is unpredictable and more apt to generate scarring.

For face and neck peeling, the chemical most preferred by facial plastic surgeons at this time is phenol, traditionally known as carbolic acid (although it is not a true acid chemically or physiologically). We would discourage you from attempting to use your knowledge of chemistry to try to influence the surgeon in his choice of chemical for your skin peeling.

I have read that the chemicals used in skin peeling can cause complications. But if I choose to have chemosurgery, what risks do I take?

The chemicals used in chemosurgery can produce multiple hypertrophic (raised) scars and ulcerations from ensuing cellulitis (infection). The scarring occurs most frequently on the chin and the neck, but it can occur in any areas where the acid has been applied.

Another serious complication is coarsening of the skin texture; the skin exhibits an orange-peel appearance similar to that seen following the healing of a deep second degree burn.

The above complications occur most frequently when diluted solutions of phenol are used instead of full strength solution and when areas of skin below the face are treated that should be avoided because of their poor regenerative powers.

When skin complications occur following skin peeling, dermal abrasion or cortone injections are attempted to soften the scarring. Surgery for true deformities caused by chemical burns may entail plastic surgical procedures such as Z-plasties and skin grafts.

Complications of kidney dysfunction can arise if the patient who has kidney pathology is treated with chemical peeling, either accidentally or deliberately. A careful history and laboratory work-up must weed out the kidney problem cases, for rapid absorption of the acid can overburden even normal kidney function and throw a patient into shock. This is one critical reason why chemosurgery must remain only in the hands of experienced medical personnel.

I would like to have my fine wrinkles removed, but I am afraid of the risks involved. What are the possible complications?

Chemical skin peeling, the procedure of choice, is least risky with patients who have blond, red, or auburn hair and blue eyes, and who want to do away with fine wrinkling of the skin. If this method is applied to other than these individuals then the risk of complications multiplies. Wise surgeons therefore refuse patients unsuitable for this procedure.

The face is the only area of the body that has reasonably good and predictable results with skin peeling. The remainder of the body skin reacts unfavorably to chemical peeling because it lacks the regenerative powers of facial skin, which is richly supplied with dermal appendage (hair follicles, sebaceous glands) from which epidermal and dermal regeneration occurs.

In contrast to the goals sought from chemical skin peeling, the face lift is calculated to get rid of excess facial skin but will do little for fine wrinkling. In many cases where there is fine wrinkling and excess facial skin, the ideal procedure is to do the face lift first followed sometime later by a chemical skin peel. Small areas of the face (like the lip area) can receive chemical peeling along with the face lift operation. The combination of both procedures can give a most outstanding result.

The procedures of chemosurgery for improvement of the appearance of the skin are now extensively practiced among plastic surgeons. The formula for the solution that is used is safe provided that it remains in the hands of physicians and that the patient's suitability has been determined by a complete general examination.

What is the most serious complication
of chemosurgery that I can encounter?

Phenol toxicity is the most serious complication of chemosurgery. This can range from renal and liver damage to poisoning of the medullary (brain) centers and cardiac muscles, which is characterized by vasomotor collapse, convulsions, respiratory failure, and ultimate death if not aggressively treated with intravenous cardiac and respiratory stimulants.

Phenol is no stranger to the human organism and when introduced into the body it is quickly detoxified and oxidized into harmless products.

Although no known toxic level of blood phenol has been established for man, we do know that the body is fully capable of handling a *small* amount of absorbed phenol when a normally functioning liver is present.

Can chemosurgery do something for my
skin that a face lift cannot do?

A face lift can smooth out deep facial wrinkles. Chemosurgery (like dermal abrasion) is unique in its ability to improve the quality and texture of the skin. Thin, fine-textured skin with shallow lines and wrinkling can usually be improved by chemosurgery. More likely you and most other people who seek elimination of the signs of aging skin will have greatest success with a face lift followed by chemosurgery where necessary. The decision of choice must be left to the judgment of your facial plastic surgeon. Some plastic surgeons say that 75 percent of their cases have chemosurgery following face lifting.

**Can chemosurgery close the large pores
on the skin of my face?**

Pores are not elastic nor is their size amenable to any method of permanent control. When the facial swelling subsides following chemical skin peeling or dermal abrasion, the pores return as vividly as ever. In fact, where there are numerous and closely packed skin pores, as on the nose and inner cheek areas, the chemical, phenol, is particularly hazardous since it is absorbed not only via the intact skin but also through the cutaneous appendages (sweat glands, hair follicles, oil glands) allowing quicker and deeper penetration than desired, with the increased possibility of injury to the skin.

**What chemical is most frequently used to
accomplish the skin peeling or chemosurgery? Would you use this chemical?**

Phenol, traditionally known as carbolic acid (although it is not a true acid chemically or physiologically), is the preferred agent for face peeling.

It is an old chemical and very dependable in the hands of the experienced physician. Essentially a keratocoagulant, in high concentration it causes rapid and complete coagulation of the surface keratin proteins, loosely combining with them to form larger molecules with new physical and chemical properties. The newly formed molecules are not absorbed through the skin as easily as free phenol, since the coagulum that is formed creates a relatively, but not absolutely, impervious barrier to phenol absorption.

When phenol is diluted, skin absorption may occur before coagulation of the surface keratin can form a perfect coagulum. Thus, dilution of the phenol enhances skin absorption and increases the danger of adverse reactions, such as scarring and systemic activity.

**Will I need general anesthesia for a
full face peeling?**

A full face peel can be done without administering any general or local anesthesia. Usually the patient is well sedated at the time of the procedure, the sedation having been started an hour or two before the operative time.

There is a minimal amount of burning sensation when the acid is applied to the skin. This sensation quickly subsides since the chemical applied for the peeling acts as a local anesthesia.

Postoperative discomfort is controlled by an analgesic (mild painkiller such as Tylenol or Darvon Plain). If the patient feels more discomfort than can be controlled by analgesics, then morphine, meperidine (Demerol), or codeine by injection is administered.

**What effects will chemosurgery have on
my skin? Actually, what is taking place
when chemicals are put on the skin?**

When the phenol is applied with cotton swabs, the skin turns white for a few minutes and then becomes swollen and red. In effect you have received a second degree burn.

About thirty minutes after application of the chemical, your face is puffy and secretes fluid. Several hours later the skin turns brown. You may feel pain for one or two hours at this stage. This pain is relieved with the use of analgesics (painkilling drugs). Pain gradually subsides.

If tape is used to increase the action of the chemical, these occlusive dressings can be removed after two days. But before peeling off the tape, the physician prescribes an analgesic. A powder containing iodides is then sprinkled on your skin, which begins to form a white, pebbly surface. The powder is repeated several times for the next two days to maintain a dry, clean area. If no adhesive tape was used, no powders are needed since the raw skin does not secrete too much fluid. Iced compresses are used around the eyes to keep down swelling, and the patient's head is kept elevated.

After about three days, a thin crust forms on the untaped face, which gradually cracks in the healing process. At this time there may be some itching. In about one week there is separation of the crusted area of the face and then there is a peeling of the surface of the cheeks, the chin, around the lips, and the forehead. In about two weeks all the crust is off the face and forehead, and you have a smooth, pinkish skin.

If the face was taped, followed by use of powder, the cake mask is removed in about one week, leaving a tight, fresh, sparkling skin. Of course, the tightness subsides somewhat when the loss of swelling brings back some of the fine wrinkles, and there is some momentary disappointment to the patient. Herein lies the moment of truth. Not *every* line of aging can be erased by any known method today. The overall effect, however, in our experience and that of our colleagues, is quite pleasing and worth the trouble.

Why do some people who have experienced chemosurgery have white blotches on their skin?

This reverse of hyperpigmentation is hypopigmentation, which is generally irreversible. Melanocytes in the epidermis have been destroyed and do not regenerate. Of course, these whitened areas can be camouflaged with makeup.

Does every face require taping after chemical peeling?

If the skin is leathery and sunbaked, taping should and can be performed with minimum risk. Thin, fine-textured skin with shallow lines and wrinkling can be improved without occlusive (taping) dressings. Taping enhances skin maceration, causing more surface damage, which increases the risk of phenol penetration and dermal scarring.

It is dangerous to tape or use a potent solution on the neck. A buffered preparation should be utilized. Even with buffered solutions, the cauterants must not be carried over the clavicle bone line. More is to be gained by peeling the neck several times with a buffered mixture than to chance scarring with an unbuffered one.

**Will the pigmented areas on my face
return after chemosurgery?**

Hyperpigmentation occasionally returns on the patient's face after several weeks or months if the patient's natural skin tone is dark, and if he has been exposed to long and intensive sun exposure. The chemicals used in chemosurgery do not change the reproductive processes of the skin since they do not reach the layers of the skin where reproduction is carried out (nor are they meant to). When the skin restores its epidermal cells after chemosurgery, these cells may contain excessive melanin, causing the hyperpigmentation to return.

**I have heard that some people's skin
turns darker after chemical peeling. Is
that a common occurrence?**

Hyperpigmentation and blotching are uncommon complications of chemosurgery provided that the plastic surgeon is careful in excluding the type of individual who would be subject to such skin changes. Chemosurgery is not indicated in patients who have darker tints of skin coloring, black hair, and brown eyes. If these individuals are excluded from those who can benefit from the chemical skin peeling procedure, then the complications of hyperpigmentation rarely occur unless the patient deliberately or nonchalantly exposes himself to the ultraviolet radiations of the sun too soon after the treatment. In the event that hyperpigmentation or blotching does occur, dermal abrasion on these patients or repeeling will generally correct these aftereffects.

cosmetic
ear
surgery

The external ears are the features of the head that we notice least on ourselves, since they are not in our direct line of vision when we look in the mirror, unless they protrude considerably beyond their normal position. Other children taunt the child whose ears protrude, and this annoyance continues into adulthood with good-natured jibes. Perhaps not taken seriously by those who do not have this problem, projecting ears are no laughing matter to their owner.

Deformities of the ear take various shapes, and cosmetic surgeons have devised some intricate techniques for making the large ear smaller, replacing missing pieces of this mazelike structure, and even totally rebuilding a missing ear.

Although hearing is not directly involved in cosmetic and reconstructive ear surgery, the external ear provides the entrance way for the sounds that must reach the middle ear. When the surgeon performs otoplastic procedures he has in mind not only cosmetic appearance but also the vital function of the ear, the transmission of sound.

Just before your child starts school, between five and seven years of age, is an ideal time to have protruding ears surgically corrected. The growth factor in the following years will not affect this surgery and the child will be saved from years of torment by other children who have the uncanny ability to pick out any abnormal feature and use it for their amusement.

Most protruding ears are cup-shaped because of the lack of the normal ear architecture. Missing is a vertical fold of cartilage, the antihelix, near the curled periphery of the ear, the helix. If you hold with thumb and forefinger the outer rim of the protruding ear of a child and force it back gently to the skull, you will see the sudden appearance of the antihelix. Most of the deformed ears for which plastic surgeons are consulted are *normal in size,* but protrude and lack the formation of this antihelix. The surgeon returns the ear to normal position and establishes the missing structure.

Cosmetic surgery for protruding ears (otoplasty) is painless and performed under general anesthesia for children and local anesthesia for adults. It scarcely incapacitates the child or adult beyond his day or two in the hospital. A dressing remains over the ears for several days, but it is not a source of discomfort. The patient must sleep in a "stocking hat" for several weeks after all dressings are removed to insure that no damage is done to the healing area.

Taking the spring from the ears by excising some of the firm cartilage from behind the ear is a well established surgical method of correction. But the most popular method of the day for otoplasty is to accordion-pleat the cartilage. This suture technique does *not* remove any of the excess cartilage but merely folds the cartilage on itself and holds the pleat (newly created antihelix) in place with sutures.

Since it is cartilage which gives the ear its skeletal structure, firmness, shape, and pliability, the plastic surgeon can quickly determine, upon examination, if his patient is suitable for the suture method of otoplasty. When examining the patient the surgeon folds the ear back upon itself into a normal position. If his fingers can fold the ear with ease, he knows the cartilage is soft and pliable enough to be suitable for suture otoplasty. If it takes force to fold and hold the ear in normal position, the surgeon can perform a modified method by shaving down and thinning out the cartilage until it is sufficiently pliable to fold upon itself.

When a patient, child or adult, is not suitable for the folding and suturing technique of otoplasty, the classical method is chosen. In this case a large section of ear cartilage is removed, permitting the surgeon to "pin" the ears back toward the skull with ease. The deformity of protruding ears is gone although the appearance of the ear may not be entirely normal because the convolution of the antihelix is missing. However, the ear is cosmetically pleasing because of normal positioning.

At what age can I have my child's protruding ears corrected by plastic surgery?

When a child is five to seven years of age, his ears have grown sufficiently large to be considered adult size and suitable for corrective surgery. The ear has assumed its full adult shape and proportion at this age and will respond to plastic surgical correction by otoplasty. Usually his cartilage, which determines the shape of his ears, is sufficiently pliable for the simpler technique of folding the cartilage back on itself and suturing it into normal position in line with the skull. The surgical correction for protruding ears at this early school age will serve him a lifetime.

As an adult is it too late to have protruding ears corrected surgically?

Correction of protruding ears is certainly not limited to children. There are probably as many adult males and females having otoplasty as children.

The adult with pliable cartilage can have the suture method, which does not excise excess protruding ear cartilage but folds it back on itself, taking care of the protrusion as well as improving the architecture of the ear.

Adults with less pliable cartilage may require the procedure which thins out the cartilage as a preliminary step in the surgery of suture technique.

The remainder of adults will have the classical technique of excising excess cartilage and suturing the ear back into a position against the head.

Even the new longer hair styles of men do not take care of the deformity of protruding ears. Males find it appalling to see the top of their ears protruding through their long hair styles.

Will taping my child's ears when he goes to bed at night help them to go back in the normal position?

Taping a child's ears at night will only keep the ears in normal position during the night and will in no way affect the position of the ears during the day. In the best interests of the child and yourself, we recommend that you follow the advice of a plastic surgeon, who would surely encourage that your child have an otoplasty for protruding ears providing he is in good general health and of the proper age. A child who develops a fully grown ear at the age of five or six can be considered a candidate for otoplasty. Plastic surgeons advise that the child's ears be placed in normal position surgically before the child attends school. The torment of other children who take innocent delight in ridiculing their playmate's defects can affect a young person's psyche for the remainder of his life.

No manipulation of the child's ears by the parents will prevent the ears from protruding from the skull. The ears are not young trees that can be made to bend or grow straight as the horticulturist would guide them by supporting devices.

I have no earlobes. My ears grow
straight against my face. Can something
be done to give me earlobes?

> The simplest method of giving you the appearance of an
> earlobe does not entail the surgical construction of ear-
> lobes. If a surgeon makes an incision at the point where
> the earlobe meets the face and carries this incision
> straight up for some millimeters in front and behind the
> earlobe, the bottom of your ear will be freed from your
> face. The pendulous portion resulting from this surgical
> procedure will be your earlobe. It is usually pendulous
> enough to hold an earring and will appear as normal a
> feature as any other person's ear.

Can my ears be made smaller in size?

> Your ears are probably smaller than you realize, but the
> fact that they protrude makes them appear unusually
> large. Most patients are completely satisfied with the
> appearance, including size of the ears, after the plastic
> surgeon has placed them close to the head in their nor-
> mal position. Allow the facial plastic surgeon to correct
> your deformity by bringing your ears closer to your
> head with the fullest expectation that you will be satis-
> fied with the result.

What is the fee for an otoplasty?

> The fee range of cosmetic ear surgery is from $750 to
> $1,500. Variations of the fee depend upon the extent of
> reconstruction, the area in which the surgeon practices,
> the experience of the surgeon, and the demand for his
> services.

I am unable to wear eyeglasses because
of a deformity of the upper one-third
of my ears. Can this condition be
corrected by ear surgery?

> Plastic surgeons have become versatile in the technique
> of reconstructing the upper one-third or one-half of the
> external ear. This deformity of the ear is corrected with

the aid of silicone implants or diced cartilage to give normal contour and strength to the upper part of the ear. Surgery to correct deformities of the upper portion of the ears will permit the use of eyeglasses, with temples straight back or angled, behind the ear.

I did amateur boxing and was punched on the ears many times. Now one ear protrudes and looks larger than the other. Can this ear have plastic surgery to make it look normal again?

The single "cauliflower" ear, a deformed ear due to irregularity of the auricular cartilage caused by trauma (injury), is a common deformity found among prize-fighters. However, it can occur to anyone who has had recurrent blows to the ear. The perichondrium (the cartilage covering) becomes thickened from subperichondrial bleeding. The result is an interruption of the normal nutrition of the cartilage, causing it to become thickened because of fibrosis that occurs with healing.

The plastic surgeon will make skin incisions into the external ear and he will attempt to place these incisions in the most inconspicuous areas so that the scars will not be obvious. After the incision is made, he will elevate the skin and subcutaneous tissue and incise the perichondrium. He will remove the thickened areas of perichondrium and cartilage which cause the deformity.

After I have surgical correction for my protruding ears, will the scars show?

Surgery for protruding ears is performed by making incisions behind the ears in the area of the natural fold of the skin. The scars heal well and cannot be seen with the naked eye.

The position of the protruding ear is changed by removing some of the stiff cartilage that holds the ear away from the head. The cartilage and skin removed are taken from the area of the major incisions behind the ear. There is no incision made in front of the ear for this corrective surgery. Visibility of the scar offers no problem, since it falls behind the ear in the groove between it and the side of the head or the mastoid region and lies hidden and unnoticed there.

Can the operation to correct ear deformity affect hearing?

Cosmetic plastic surgery for ear deformities, such as protruding ears, in no way affects the hearing of the patient. The hearing centers, including the auditory nerve, are deep within the aural cavity and the brain. The area of surgery for ear deformity is shallow by comparison.

Are there any serious complications that can occur in cosmetic ear surgery?

Although this is usually a successful operation, there have been complications faced by plastic surgeons in this field.

This part of the body has a meager blood supply, which can be a source of trouble. A lack of blood supply to the portion of the ear that has been incised and separated in part from the head becomes a potential source of infection. Total loss of blood supply to the ear can cause atrophy and destruction of the ear. A too-tight dressing has been known to cause this disaster, necessitating a series of complicated operations for reconstruction of a new ear.

Fortunately this complication of loss of blood supply is rare and plastic surgery for correction of ear deformities is a source of happy improvement for the youngster (or adult) who has this defect.

How long after my ear operation will I be able to resume wearing my eyeglasses?

Because the technique used most frequently today does not place the ear back too closely against the head, and, because there is now a normal amount of space behind the ear by the use of a suture technique of otoplasty, the patient may wear his eyeglasses within three weeks after surgery. During the period of wearing the dressing, the temples of the eyeglasses can be adjusted or temporarily replaced to fit straight back instead of bending behind the ear. After dressings have been removed, straight temples can be worn for another two weeks. With children, and some adults, an athletic headband can be attached to the ends of the temples to maintain the eyeglasses snugly against the head.

How soon after my ear surgery can I have my ears pierced?

Following the suture technique otoplasty, healing will be sufficient to allow piercing of the earlobes after one month. A surgeon who knows the desires of the patient about ear piercing in advance may accommodate by piercing the lobes at the time of surgery and maintaining the opening with a ringlike suture until a gold earring can be worn.

Anatomy of the external ear

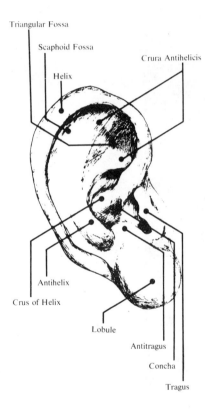

Triangular Fossa

Scaphoid Fossa

Crura Antihelicis

Helix

Antihelix

Crus of Helix

Lobule

Antitragus

Concha

Tragus

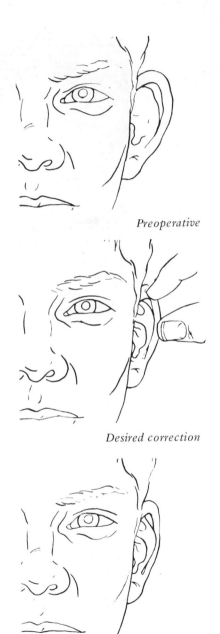

Preoperative

Desired correction

Postoperative

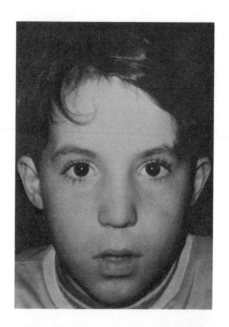

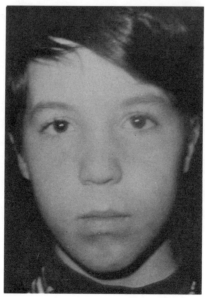

Otoplasty for protruding ears

hair
transplantation

Baldness in men has been accepted by the women of the world with no diminution of respect or love for the male. The male with baldness, however, has not been so tolerant of his own physical defect. Over the centuries he has borne his disfigurement with unhappy stoicism, always seeking a miracle drug or ointment that would reawaken the dead hair follicles. But reawakening the dead has escaped every manner of prayer and intellectual gymnastic. It was apparent that the male of the species had no recourse for this painless but pathetic cosmetic defect, except a hair piece when baldness too greatly offended his vanity or his income, if a career was at stake.

Hair transplantation, a surgical technique of transferring hairgrowing follicles in a bed of skin and underlying tissue from the fertile area of the scalp to the infertile denuded area, is the first breakthrough in this never-ending quest for a socially acceptable male head of hair.

The technique of hair transplantation is a highly specialized cosmetic surgical skill that has proven to be successful to the extent that the hair is truly transplanted and grows. The limitation lies in the length of time involved to transplant a reasonably large enough number of hair plugs to suggest a natural head of hair. A full head of hair may have up to 100,000 hairs, whereas the transplanted head has only a rearrangement of the existing hairs to satisfy a normal hair pattern. But like all limitations in reaching a desired goal, plateaus along the way provide satisfaction for those willing to make the struggle.

As with the problem of rejection of transplanted organs, the transplanted hair from another donor has not proven successful. Until medical research provides us with the means of inhibiting the production of antibodies which cause body rejection of donor transplants, we cannot start a "hair bank" nor can you accept the kind offers of a hairy relative or friend. It is fascinating to contemplate the future possibility of transplanting hair from the amply supplied female head to the impoverished male head!

Since the patient provides his own source of transplanted hair, he must have an ample growth in the back of the scalp (occipital) and sides of the scalp (temporal). If these areas are already sparse, the source has dried up. The benefits derived, if any, will not be worth the time, discomfort, and cost involved. If "fuzz" is more attractive to the patient than a totally bald pate, there is some justification for the transplant procedure. Also, a frontal transplanted hairline may help to mask a hair piece, just as with women's wigs and wiglets, a combing of the woman's own front hairs over the wig disguises it.

There can be troubles along the way even in the most ideal patient, that is, the patient who has a healthy and ample supply of peripheral hair. At times, whether out of biological perversity or a surgeon's unfamiliarity with the procedure, the newly planted hair does not "take." The punch hole remaining will, of course, leave a small scar. Attempts can be made to replant new beds of hair follicle in close proximity to the unsuccessful plug so that a "take" will eventually cover the residual scar. When all attempts fail, the hair piece is always available to cover the bald head along with the "trial and errors."

Hair transplantation, a relatively new technique in the field of cosmetic surgery, is continuing to gain increased acceptance by the medical profession and the public as experimentation improves technique. Not many individuals volunteer to be "guinea pigs," but this field, like others in modern cosmetic facial plastic surgery, is new enough to demand a certain spirit of adventure and bravado on the part of the patient.

If I am willing to pay a double fee
can larger plugs be transplanted at
each session to hasten the procedures?

The size of the plugs of hair follicles transplanted appears to be in direct proportion to the success of the procedure. The plugs that are larger than those considered to be normal, about four millimeters, have a much lower survival rate. Rather than run the risk of failure of "takes" with resultant scars, it would be more judicious to allow the surgeon to use the smaller plugs and wait patiently for the gradual build up of clusters of hair plugs.

I am only twenty-two years of age and
I am already losing hair. Can I start
my hair transplantation now and expect
to have better results than if I wait
until a later age?

Plastic surgeons are frequently consulted by individuals who become terrified at the first awareness of hair loss. We see many young people with this condition and many of them appear to have a full head of hair despite their complaint. It is only when the patient points out to the surgeon the extent of the recession and where the recession is apparent to him that the surgeon can evaluate the alleged loss. If your condition does not strike the surgeon immediately as a cosmetic deformity of some importance that needs correction, he will hardly recommend that you undergo surgery for it. If the extent of loss of hair were obvious it would be immediately recognized by the surgeon that you are consulting, because of early baldness or receding hairline. Often the balding surgeon who is consulted would be overjoyed to have one-half the amount of hair that many of his patients have who request hair transplants.

During hair transplantation can a hair piece be worn or will it interfere with new transplanted hair growth?

During the first week after transplantation no hair piece should be worn. When the scalp looks as though it is well healed, all crust formation is gone, and there is no evidence of any separation between donor plugs of hair and skin to recipient areas (complete closure of punch graft holes), then it is safe to wear your hairpiece.

Is hair transplantation painful?

Hair transplantation should not be painful since the areas where the surgeon works—both donor (back of head) and recipient (front of scalp receiving the plugs)—are well anesthetized with injections of a local anesthetic.

During the healing period in the days to follow, there may be some discomfort, and this is alleviated by pain-relieving medication taken by mouth at regular intervals. A sedative can be taken at bed time if you are restless and irritable due to your discomfort. This period of mild pain passes in several days. You are ready for your next session of hair transplantation in about four to six weeks.

How is the hair transplanted from the back of my head to the bald area?

The surgeon uses a trephine, a surgical instrument which is about three to four millimeters in diameter, has a sharp round cutting edge, and looks like a miniature cookie cutter. Before removal of the plugs, the hair is trimmed close to the scalp. Under local anesthesia injected into the scalp at the back of the head where the hair is most luxuriant, the plugs are removed from this donor area and placed in a sterile glass dish. A technician trims the plugs to remove extraneous tissue, but he takes care not to injure any of the hair follicles.

The area to receive the graft (recipient area), which has also been prepared for surgery by sterilization and anesthesia with procaine (Novocaine), will have plugs of scalp removed by the same instrument, so that the hair plugs prepared by the technician can be inserted with great ease. Attention is paid to the direction of the normal hair growth in each plug so that when the hair emerges, it grows in the proper direction. No matter how anxious you are to have a good head of hair, you would not be happy to have it continually growing down over your eyes. All plugs are kept in place by pressure dressings which are removed within three to four days.

How many hairs are transplanted at each surgical session?

You will have about twenty to thirty plugs with hair transplanted at each surgical procedure performed in the doctor's office. Each plug of scalp has about fifteen to twenty hair shafts. The greater the hair density found in the donor area the more optimistic one can be about the future growth of eventual hair shafts that makes the hair transplantation successful. A "crash" job is inadvisable because the plugs must not be too large for a "take." Besides, the patient and surgeon cannot endure too long a session. Each plug requires care in removal, trimming, and insertion. The average safe size for each plug is about three to four millimeters. When the plugs are kept to this size, the "takes" are mostly successful.

**Is there any fast way to have
hair transplanted?**

If you are a young person who has lost hair prematurely, you are a candidate for a procedure called strip grafts. Several sections of scalp, one-fourth inch in width and about four inches long, are taken from the full-hair section in the back of the head and transplanted to the balded area. If the strips take, you may have other sets of strips transplanted in about three weeks. The wounds in the donor area are sutured without evidence of scarring or disturbance of the hair follicles. The strip is sutured into place in the nude area. This procedure can be done in the office, but might be more comfortably and safely performed in the hospital.

If the surgeon decides that a large graft will be attempted, he can perform it by swinging a pedicle graft (skin and hair) and thereby maintaining the blood supply, because one end of the graft is still attached to its original site. After several weeks the attached skin is severed from its home site and sutured into its new location.

**What is the plan that the plastic
surgeon has in mind for the "bald"
person having hair transplantation?**

Your plastic surgeon or the dermatologist who does this type of surgery will plan to first create a frontal hairline with a normal looking pattern of widow's peak. The first plugs of hair (numbering about twenty to thirty plugs) are spaced evenly in the general design. Future sessions continue the filling in of this front section so that the hair can gain a fuller look by combining the longer hairs that have grown since the previous transplant with the newly placed plugs of hair. The plan is to continue to fill in from the front toward the back.

What is the fee for hair transplantation?

Most surgeons charge by the number of hair plugs transplanted, five to ten dollars per plug. The patient can have about twenty-five plugs per session. Some surgeons will undertake to transplant fifty and more plugs in one session, with the consent of the patient. The fee would range accordingly.

Does transplantation increase the number of hairs on the head?

Hair transplantation does not increase the number of hairs on the head, but merely rearranges them in a more pleasing pattern. The more abundantly endowed donor sites in the back of the scalp give up some of their plenty to the bare or sparsely furnished frontal area in order to restore a vanishing hairline or a circle of bare crown. The donor site heals as a hairless scar. However, since the hairs grow so close together in the back and sides of the head, the donor site is hidden in the "forest." The new plugs of hair, usually numbering about a dozen individual hairs, lose their original hairs in the new setting and grow fresh hairs in several weeks, but always no more than the same number as in the original plug graft and sometimes fewer.

My husband is satisfied with his hair transplants and I would like to have the same procedure for my receding hairline. Can a woman have hair transplanted?

There is no difference in the biological response in hair transplantation between men and women. The hair transplants are taken from the back of the head where there is an ample supply of hair. The hair plugs are placed in the sparse area in the front of the head where the area has been properly prepared by the removal of similar sized plugs in order to receive the new hair plugs. Up to twenty-five plugs can be transplanted at one sitting. The newly transplanted plugs of hair and scalp require that they be placed so that the new growth of hair will grow in the proper direction. If the hair transplants are used to create a hairline, the surgeon must pay careful attention to this feature.

Before women are accepted for hair transplantation, the plastic surgeon may suggest a consultation with an internist or endocrinologist to explore the possibilities of endocrine insufficiency or other possible medical complications. Successful medical treatment of a condition responsible for female hair loss may restore hair through the normal regrowth processes. Female hair loss does not parallel in origin male hair loss and therefore cannot be evaluated in the same manner.

I am a woman who has always envied a widow's peak. Can I have hair transplanted to attain this feature?

Any plastic surgeon would say to this patient that if she has a normal hairline she should do nothing to change her appearance that would require surgery. The newly formed hairline might eventually enhance a female's appearance, but not sufficiently so to run the risk involved with the possibility of scar formation if hair plugs are lost. Scars can also form around the hair plug even if successfully transplanted. If the threat of scarring could be totally eliminated, this request for a widow's peak could easily be fulfilled.

Will all the hair follicles transplanted from the back area of my head "take" in their new location in the bald area?

There has been sufficient experimentation and successful practice by plastic surgeons and dermatologists in the field of hair transplantation to assure the skeptical prospective patient that this is a bona fide and well regarded technique of hair restoration to bald areas of the scalp. Actually, there is an almost 100 percent take of plugs of hair transplanted when handled by experienced medical men. However, in each plug there are about fifteen to twenty hair shafts and follicles, and if the full complement of hair follicles do not sprout, at least 50 percent or more will begin to appear. The overall acceptance of the recipient area of the scalp to the transplanted hair is most remarkable.

How long will it take to give me a
full head of hair?

The expectation of quickly restoring a bald head to a full head of hair belongs in never, never land. The normal full head of hair is so luxuriant in number of hairs that it would take several hundred visits to the surgeon's office to equal it. Some men are persistent and continue transplantation treatments indefinitely, always striving for perfection. Other men are perfectly satisfied with some hair restored to what was formerly a bald area. To cover the average baldness of a man adequately would take somewhere between twenty to fifty surgical procedures.

Does the hair restore itself where it
is removed to provide the
transplanted plug?

The hair plug, containing the hair follicle, skin, and some subcutaneous tissue, does not leave a source of restoration at the donor site. The surgeon is merely moving the "potted plant" from one side of the patio to the other. The donor site heals, leaving a faint scar that will not be noticeable because of the surrounding hair growing over it.

I am a tennis pro and would like to
know if I would be incapacitated for a
long period of time while undergoing
hair transplantation?

Hair transplants require nourishment through blood supply, and proper dressings are needed during the healing period. The newly placed hair transplants are not sutured into their positions and, therefore, require a period of about three weeks to become permanently fixed.

The donor site, from which the plugs have been taken, occasionally bleeds sufficiently to require hemostasis (control of bleeding) by suturing. The majority of donor sites do not need suturing for closure. To permit proper healing, it is advisable that no exertion should be permitted for several weeks following surgery. You, as a tennis professional, should choose the time of year that would allow you sufficient time for rest and permit you to refrain from vigorous activities like tennis.

Hair transplant

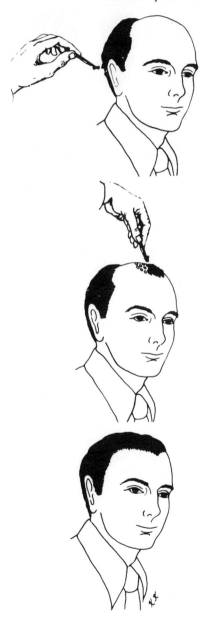

correction
of scars

Scars of the face from traumatic injury or disease may involve only the skin, but their effect may reach the heart and mind of the scarred patient. There is no way to measure the damage caused by what is seen on the surface. External healing often masks the real wound—a deep despair and sorrow over the loss of one's normal facial appearance.

Facial plastic surgery is indeed necessary for repairs of scars and deformities caused by injuries. Although every scar removal usually provides some improvement in the cosmetic appearance, the excised scar will be replaced by another scar. Fortunately the new scar is usually less conspicuous. The surgeon plans his operation for scar removal with infinite care for the details of the texture and direction of muscle layers. He will obtain the best results if the scar can be removed and the wound margins brought together without tension. If the scar is wide and irregular, he may choose a series of operations removing more sections of the scar with each procedure, until all of the old scar is removed and just the fine line of the last remaining scar can be seen.

When the scar is so large and irregular that excising it even by a series of operations would not be satisfactory, a graft of skin from a donor area is planned. The choice of method of removal must be left to your surgeon.

Surgery can often be assisted by radiotherapy (X-ray), dermal abrasion, and chemosurgery in obtaining postoperative improvement of the scar. Newly formed scar tissue responds well to X-ray therapy, which can limit its growth. After a second or third excision, dermal abrasion will refine the scar even further if necessary.

The location of the scar influences its healing and resultant appearance. A scar located in mobile tissue as in the cheek is more difficult to repair than one located on a firm base such as the forehead or nose. Horizontal scars on the eyelids leave an imperceptible line.

Children and young adults are more likely to develop wide, overgrown scars even though they heal more rapidly. The shape of a scar influences the result after surgical removal. Semicircular or U-shaped scars are more difficult to improve than a less curved or jagged scar. However, multiple excisions over a period of time will surely provide cosmetic improvement.

There are disappointments for both the patient and the surgeon along the path of facial plastic and reconstructive surgery for scars. Hopes are often too high for dramatic results that are impossible to achieve. A well-planned course of surgical correction is usually discussed by the surgeon and his patient so that there will be a better understanding of what is expected and what lies ahead. The plastic surgeon's ability to accurately excise the old scar, undermine the skin, and approximate the new skin edges affords you the best opportunity for cosmetic improvement of facial scars.

In making a fine hairline scar from a scar that has caused deformity and needs revision, a technique has been devised which avoids the usual straight-line incision but utilizes an interdigital (interlocking toothlike) incision. These irregular or staggered incision lines are being performed by plastic surgeons who claim great success in obtaining an inconspicuous scar.

Radiotherapy (X-ray therapy) is used by plastic surgeons if the surgeon is concerned with postoperative healing. Some patients have a tendency to overheal and to develop a hypertrophied scar which can be thick and elevated above the normal surface of the skin. These scars remain red in color for several months. Radiotherapy applies a roentgen-ray burn to the skin in measured degrees on the newly formed capillaries and fibrous tissue. The aim of this therapy is to restrain the growth factors and prevent overgrowth of the healed scar.

To avoid hypertrophied scarring, or keloids, the plastic surgeon will recommend the patient to have X-ray therapy within a few days following surgery. A series of X-ray treatments might be just enough to prevent a hypertrophied scar. Radiotherapy is avoided in treating scars of the nose and ears since it can cause a deformity of the cartilage in both places.

The cost of plastic surgical repair of scars depends upon the size and location of the scar and degree of distortion. Scars associated with distortion require technical revision with Z-plasties or multiple Z-plasties. Fees for scar revision of this type will be higher than those for less complicated scar excision. Fees for surgical repair of scars of the face will range from $250 for a simple excision, to $1,000 or $1,500 for a complicated depressed, raised, or irregular scar that causes a deformity of the eyelids, nose, or lips. Scars of the body, neck, and extremities may call for fees of $250 to $1,000 depending upon loss of function as well as cosmetic problem.

Scars of the neck due to burns are difficult to handle, especially if the head is restricted in motion. These scars will need Z-plasties and skin transplantations and require successive procedures in most cases. Each operative procedure will usually be billed separately since each will require a separate hospital admission with several hours of operating time.

I have recently been in an accident and have an unsightly scar. Is this the time to have it removed?

Removal of a scar following injury should be deferred for several months until there is a total contraction and the skin is white and soft. Often a scar heals so well, if given enough time, that plastic surgery may no longer be required. For example, a scar may appear red and overgrown six weeks after an accident. However, if the surgeon waits six months, the scar may appear quite different. In the healing the redness will subside because the blood vessels have been squeezed dry by the healing process of fibrosis. The scar will appear smaller because of contracture of the scar tissue. As a rule, time is in your favor and no hasty decision should be made concerning scar revision until complete healing takes place.

I have a raised scar. Can this be removed without my new scar healing in the same manner?

You have a hypertrophied scar which is a result of a variation of the healing process. The scar tissue has overgrown and caused a raised scar line. This type of scar may be the result of infection of the original wound or hasty emergency suturing at the time of injury. There is every reason to believe surgical removal will be successful and that you will have a fine line scar instead of an unattractive hypertrophied scar.

In contrast to the hypertrophied scar which is usually successfully removed with surgery, there is a keloidal scar that can defy the most careful surgery and reappear. The keloidal scar is irregular, reddish, hard, and fibrous, and it can continue to grow for many months beyond normal healing time. The use of cor-tones and radiotherapy has been successful in retarding the growth of keloids.

**I have been told that because I have
dark skin my scar formed a keloid and
surgery will not help me. Is this true?**

Persons with dark skin coloring are prone to the over-production of a peculiar form of scar tissue which we call a keloid. This genetic factor makes scar removal a risk. A recurrence is likely but not absolutely assured.

A study of other scars on your body would be helpful, and the consideration of radiotherapy or cortone drugs immediately after surgery would be useful in preventing the formation of further growth of the keloid.

**Because of his growth years ahead, should
a child have plastic surgical correction
for scars delayed?**

Scars can be removed from the face of a growing child and have no bearing on the continued growth of the facial features. The youthful elasticity of the skin provides normal positioning of the skin and underlying tissues as the scar heals and growth continues.

Children find scars distressing because of the humiliation suffered by the criticism of other children. The correction of the scars, therefore, should not be delayed unnecessarily. If possible, cosmetic correction of scars should be performed before the child enters school.

Pretending to ignore the child's scars may temporarily allay his fears of being deformed, but he will soon be reminded of any disfigurement by the teasing of playmates. He may hide his anxiety from you in words but it will be manifested in other ways. If surgery is necessarily delayed the reason might better be explained briefly, tenderly, and logically to the child.

**Is there any way of predicting how
successfully a scar can be
corrected surgically?**

To predict a result in scar surgery is to tread on dangerous ground because disappointment can be so crushing to the scarred individual. If the deeper structures have not been involved—if the tendons, ligaments, nerves, and major blood vessels have not been severed—function will be restored and appearance greatly improved following plastic surgery for scars.

An important factor influencing healing of a scar is the condition of the skin edges prior to corrective surgery. If the wound is jagged and there has been considerable loss of tissue, the approximation (joining together) of the edges of the wound becomes more difficult and results are more questionable, cosmetically speaking. Of course, the skin edges are trimmed precisely, and with infinite attention paid to obtaining the smallest scar line possible, but the limitation involved is the amount of skin that can be trimmed to obtain a closure without tension.

The plastic surgeon is ready to handle the repair of a scar in whatever manner the condition requires, including the intricate steps of scar repair involving rotation flaps and skin grafts. In general the less grotesque the scar, the less surgery is required and the more predictably successful the surgery will be.

What happens to a serious laceration of the skin from an accidental injury that is allowed to heal of its own accord?

A laceration permitted to heal spontaneously will heal from the bottom up because there was no approximation of skin tissue (surgically joining the skin edges.) This usually results in a large, ugly scar that is prone to reopening upon the application of tension since the scar is extremely weak. There would probably be a great amount of redness in the region of the scar persisting for many months and in some instances never disappearing. The scar would appear irregular with the "hills and valleys" of haphazard reparative processes.

The unattended wound may never heal properly because foreign material could be present in the wound, causing constant drainage from infection. Blood clots not washed out of a wound create a source of bacterial growth. Uncontrolled infection in a wound can lead to bacteremia and septicemia (blood poisoning).

Treatment of certain wounds as those caused by objects exposed to the elements requires giving the body extra protection against the invading tetanus germs, which cause lockjaw; an injection for immunization of the body against tetanus organisms would be imperative in all such injuries.

A plastic surgeon need not attend the injured person to avoid the complications of serious lacerations, but it is vitally important that the injured patient receive skilled surgical care as quickly as possible.

How can my scar be removed and the remaining skin brought together?

A scar is excised and the skin edges are brought together without any tension. The method used is one of undermining the surrounding skin (loosening it from its subcutaneous tissue) and advancing or stretching it over the exposed area. There is a limit of stretch determined by the elasticity of the skin and the presence of sufficient blood supply. Here the judgment of the plastic surgeon is all important. If these basic principles are adhered to, you can expect a fine hairline scar.

Can a scar ever be entirely eliminated?

No incision into the skin, made accidentally by injury or purposefully by a surgeon, ever entirely "disappears." But the skilled surgeon places the scar in the natural fold of the skin, which will hide a thin scar. In accidental injury the chances of a laceration occurring in such a natural fold are no better than the odds of winning at roulette.

Facial plastic surgery affords perhaps the only opportunity for a patient to acquire scars which are un-noticeable. Because incisions are made along natural folds in the facial skin and eyelids, the scars of face lift and cosmetic eyelid surgery are rarely seen.

Is it possible for a surgical incision for cosmetic plastic surgery to defy healing and leave the patient with an unattractive scar?

An incision may not heal because the patient did not receive the necessary preoperative care that would reveal by laboratory testing that he or she had a medical condition such as diabetes, blood dyscrasia, venereal disease, or poor nutrition. An adequate history and physical examination are important to seek out information that indicates surgical complications like poor healing of a surgical incision.

Local infections of incisions can also occur from the presence of bacterial organisms in the air and all about us, even when all precautions are taken to maintain asepsis during and after surgery. Normally these bacterial infections are overcome easily and promptly with antibiotics. If the infection persists, the offending organisms are identified with the aid of culture testing in a laboratory and they are then attacked by the specific antibiotics to which they are most sensitive. There is little likelihood that adequate treatment would not eventually conquer an infection and permit the incision to heal properly.

cosmetic breast surgery

The generously endowed bosom has not always been in fashion in our culture. Its ups and downs—from prominence to oblivion—have intrigued fashion designers, male admirers, artists, and writers for many centuries. Every culture differs in its emphasis on the human female breast, some celebrating it, some ignoring it, but all cultures, even those with dominant male chauvinism, have given credit to the female body where credit was due: the woman's body performs nature's mightiest task—the bearing of a child, with the breasts doing the wonder of wonders, providing nourishment and psychological support to the newborn.

Woman should indeed be proud of her beautiful torso so idealized for centuries by Greek sculptors, Renaissance artists and poets, and even contemporary Pop artists.

Defeminizing forces have hidden the female breast from view from time to time behind a facade of religious decorum or puritanical denial of the physical form. Primitive cultures have seldom resorted to this unnatural posture concerning the female anatomy. The youth revolt frees the female from the restraints of conservative fashion mores, as with the modern style of the braless look and partial breast exposure. This new feminine trend, au naturelle, has encouraged women to accept their bodies as offered by nature.

On the other extreme, permissiveness in display of the sex symbols and sex acts in the arts has encouraged an overemphasis of the female body, and in particular, the female breast. Many women of today feel obliged to present a full-breasted figure to compete with the apparent male interest in the generous-sized female breast.

The physical development of the female breast starts at puberty between the ages of eleven and thirteen. The developed female breast is composed of skin, subcutaneous tissue, fat, and mammary gland tissue with lactiferous ducts leading to the nipple. When the breast fails to develop to maturity during puberty, the glandular tissue is scant or absent.

When the female reaches age sixteen to eighteen and she has not developed a full, round breast, she is instinctively concerned about her appearance. Looking around her, she sees other women whose breast projection is obvious, and she feels denied the most important evidence of her female adulthood. Although greatly disappointed and often emotionally disturbed about this, she is usually inhibited in vocalizing this distress to her parents or friends. Unfortunately, her concern for her inadequacy is frequently misjudged, since her breast development may be quite adequate to please the male ideal of this female organ of beauty. Her resort to unnatural, fruitless, and expensive contrivances for increasing breast development is pitiful if not dangerous. No artificial manipulation with or without the use of drug items should be attempted on the female breast.

In later adult years, the breast shows the evidence of aging, when its glandular tissue and fat loss causes the breasts to appear atrophied and pendulous. At this time in life, the woman may be facing other emotional problems, normal to female life, and the added loss of beauty of face and figure, as exemplified most typically in the breast formation, leaves her with a sense of inferiority. She looks at the young body and yearns increasingly for rejuvenation. This woman, too, is the target for unsubstantiated claims concerning devices with expensive price tags that would restore her breasts to youthful fullness and projection.

Surgical restructuring of the female breast is a relatively modern technique in the history of cosmetic plastic and reconstructive surgery. In the earlier decades of this century, reconstructive breast surgery was performed for the oversized breast. Women, whether for cosmetic reasons or for physical stress of back strain resulting from excess weight, sought relief by plastic surgery.

In the technique of breast reduction, still performed routinely today, a circumareolar incision is made. Skin, subcutaneous fat, and breast tissue are then removed, sufficiently to provide a breast of normal proportions. In most cases, the nipple need not be removed and repositioned. Where the breast is unusually oversized, the nipple is isolated and repositioned. Well-documented as successful procedures, the mammaplasty (for women) and gynecoplasty (for men with abnormal amount of breast tissue) are common operations in the field of reconstructive plastic surgery.

With the development of the mammary prosthesis implants in medical science laboratories, in the form of silicones, the breast operation for enlargement, or augmentation, became a procedure readily acceptable to the plastic surgeon for its safety and its effectiveness. The silicone implant is a silicone rubber envelope filled with silicone gel, and it is inserted readily into a pocket beneath the natural breast. An incision placed inconspicuously on or near the breast fold is the opening to the pocket.

We have the chemists to thank for making this surgical technique possible. The nature of the silicone product itself provides the safety and the durability of the breast implant.

Fees for the various types of cosmetic breast surgery fall in the following ranges: reduction mammaplasty, $2,500 to $3,500; correction of gynecoplasty, $1,000 to $2,000; and breast augmentation, $750 to $2,000.

Could breast augmentation surgery have any bearing on the menopause?

Breast augmentation surgery will not hasten or delay the menopause. With menopause, breast tissue and fat become absorbed and there is less fullness of the breasts. A woman may feel more unattractive and undesirable at this time. She can improve her appearance and morale by having plastic surgery restore her youthful appearance and body contour. The surgical procedure of breast augmentation is considered safe, effective and, in many instances, a necessity for the woman who might develop a psychological fixation about the loss of her youthful appearance.

Can liquid silicone be used for breast augmentation?

Liquid silicone is no longer used for breast augmentation. After a long initial experimentation stage, liquid silicone has been found to stray from its original location, traveling to the more dependent areas of the body. Occasionally, the material has appeared in a patient's lungs or other vital organs. Because of these characteristics, liquid silicone has been abandoned and preformed silicone implants are used as a safer and more desirable method of breast augmentation.

Can I choose the size of silicone implant I want in order to have the size bosom I would like? I am a brassiere size 32-A. Can I become a 36-C with silicone implants?

The surgeon has available several sizes of breast implants. The size you seek can be discussed frankly with your surgeon. You, like many patients, may desire a breast size larger than you should expect, which is understandable as a psychological overcompensation. However the surgeon knows what size is suitable since he has already evaluated your figure in relation to the implant. He has surgical factors to consider as well. He will want to avoid pressure points which can cause over-stretching of the skin and result in a large, unattractive scar because of tension. The selection of size will be made that will please you and assure the surgeon of attaining a safe and good result. After silicone implantation, patients are several brassiere sizes larger.

Is the skin strained in stretching to cover the breast implant? If so, could this cause any discomfort or damage to the skin?

The skin of the breast, if stretched too greatly by the silicone implants, can be damaged and permanently scarred. Necrosis (death of tissue) can occur if too much pressure is placed on stretched skin and blood supply to the skin cut off or diminished by poor nourishment. Surgeons do not use a silicone breast prosthesis so large that it causes undue tension on the skin and blood vessels. Mild sensation of chest pressure postoperatively is normal. However, if pain, swelling, and redness of the skin of the breast occur at any time postoperatively, you must consult your surgeon at once.

Does breast augmentation have to be performed in a hospital? If so, how long a time of hospitalization is required?

Breast augmentation is major surgery and as such is best performed in a hospital, which provides greater sterility and greater safety in anesthesia administration. With office surgery there is great risk of possible toxic reaction from excessive local anesthesia administered, of lack of availability of resuscitative equipment, and of the additional hazard of contamination of the prosthetic implant as well as the surgical instrumentation. To insure safer surgery and the best cosmetic result, breast augmentation plastic surgery should be performed in a hospital operating room.

The usual length of hospital stay is three or four days.

**If I decide to submit to a reconstruc-
tion of my amputated breast, can I
expect my new breast to be the same size
as my normal breast?**

There are severe limitations in the ability of the surgeon to choose a proper breast size when planning a total reconstruction following amputation. The tautness of the skin of the chest wall inhibits resiliency, so a small size gel-filled prosthesis is usually chosen by the plastic surgeon. Even more suitable would probably be an inflatable prosthesis. This is a contoured silicone envelope that is inserted under the newly grafted skin and areola with nipple. The inflatable prosthesis is filled with saline (salt water) solution after insertion. A self-sealing valve encloses the saline solution in the silicone bag. The prosthesis is usually underfilled to give the new breast resiliency.

As encouraging as are the results of breast reconstruction today, there is much room for product research and development. This is going on both privately and under the direction of federal research grant programs.

**Is there a breast implant that can be
placed under the skin and inflated
which can make my breast as large as
I choose to have it?**

Inflatable breast implants made of silicone envelopes can be inserted under the breast tissue through an opening made surgically in the areola (nipple area) or through an incision in the mammary fold, the natural fold under the breast. The surgeon develops space be-

hind the breast tissue that will accommodate this prosthesis when it is filled. These envelopes can be filled
through a tube attached to the silicone bag into which is
inserted saline solution (salt water). A valve closure is
designed to prevent leakage of the saline solution. Because of the nature of this inflatable bag, the prosthesis
can be filled to suit the surgeon and patient as to size.

The inflatable implant is ideal for women who have
unequally sized breasts. It is also not difficult for the
surgeon to increase or decrease the size of the breast
with additional or less saline solution at a later date.
This would be done by making a simple incision in the
region of the valve, exteriorizing the valve, and then
making an adjustment to the size desired.

Some disadvantages of this type of breast implant
should be noted. There is frequent leakage of the saline
through the valve. Also some breasts are found to be too
hard because the silicone envelope of the inflatable prosthesis is not as soft and elastic as the gel-filled sealed
silicone prosthesis (noninflatable type). To overcome
this disadvantage, the inflatable envelopes are usually
underfilled, which allows for more resiliency when
palpated.

I have undergone a radical mastectomy
for a cancerous tumor of the breast and
I feel very depressed over my deformity.
Can a plastic surgeon help me by recon-
structing a new breast? I do not
expect perfection.

Although radical mastectomy has become less radical in
the past five years and consequently large deformities of
the axilla (underarm) and below the clavicle (collarbone) are fewer, there are still many classical radical
mastectomies being performed. The radical mastectomy
of your type has been performed because of the evidence or strong possibility of the invasion by the tumor
cells into the lymph nodes and perhaps into the retro-

mammary tissue or through the connective tissue into the nipple and surrounding. Since this type of invasion of the tumor is found in perhaps 50 percent of the cases requiring breast mastectomy, you can understand why the surgeon will use caution in performing the radical mastectomy in preference to the simple mastectomy. In fact, the patient who has had radical mastectomy will usually be required to have follow-up therapy, such as radiation (X-ray), hormones, or cobalt treatment. So it is not only the effect of the radical mastectomy but also the effects of follow-up therapy that determine the condition of the area that would require the breast reconstruction. A waiting period is necessary between the mastectomy and any contemplated attempt to reconstruct a new breast.

The surgeon who decides to undertake the reconstruction of a breast following mastectomy faces an arduous task. He must obtain sufficient skin from other parts of the body to cover the new breast and he must reconstruct the axillary area, which would require removal of dense scar tissue and resurfacing of the area with a supple skin. Silicone implant can be of aid in the reconstruction. Then there is the challenge of a satisfactory cosmetic nipple, which would need to be made from mucous membrane found in various cavities of the body such as the mouth or vagina. There is presently a technique being used of grafting the patient's own areola and nipple to the lower part of the chest during the mastectomy to protect it from the postoperative treatment (as, for instance, radiation) and to save it for future reconstruction. This procedure is only performed in rare and highly selected cases. This matter is usually discussed with the patient prior to the mastectomy.

As you can well imagine, there are complications and uncertain results in these techniques of breast reconstructive surgery. The problem of loss of suppleness of the skin following intense X-ray treatment may make reconstruction impossible because of the wide area of thin, scarred skin. A skin transplant would be out of the question in these cases.

To improve the inconsistent results of this complicated reconstructive plastic surgery, research is constant in the field of breast reconstruction. General surgeons and plastic surgeons are cooperating to develop surgical procedures to perform a radical mastectomy and reconstructive breast surgery in a one-stage operation for the patient who shows no evidence of metastasis to other critical areas of the body.

Present estimated fees for reconstructive breast surgery following radical mastectomy range from $3,500 to $5,000.

I had liquid silicone injected in my breasts several years ago. Lately I have read some very frightening stories about what has happened to women who had silicone injections. Can I have the liquid silicone removed?

To attempt removal of liquid silicone from the breast is difficult since much of the material has probably been dispersed from the site of injection and has settled in neighboring areas and dependent portions of the body. *Medical grade* liquid silicone is an inert substance and tissue reaction would therefore not occur. Most documented cases of ill effects and serious complications from liquid silicone injections reveal that *industrial grade* or *impure quality* liquid silicone was used. The Federal Food and Drug Administration has been the watchdog over silicone permitted to be used in this country and has assured those patients who received injections on an experimental basis within a controlled research program that they have been injected with only pure medical grade liquid silicone.

If there should be breast tissue reaction with infection from the injected silicone, the surgeon can remove this infected tissue along with the liquid silicone that is still present in the breast. After the infection is cleared up and the breast tissue appears normal again, a silicone implant can be used to augment the breast and restore good contour.

I know that silicone implants are used to enlarge the breast, but I am interested in lifting my sagging breasts. Can silicone implants be used for this purpose?

Abnormally small breasts that are sagging can be enlarged and made to appear higher and firmer with gel-filled silicone implants. If the breast is long and loose, perhaps because of excessive weight loss or unusual breakdown of ligaments due to improper breast support, recurrent pregnancies, or aging, another operative approach to correction is taken. An operation is performed to elevate the glandular and fatty breast tissue and to excise superfluous skin. This may be all that is necessary to give the breast proper size, shape, and form. If the end result is that the breast is too small after the surgery, a silicone implant can be inserted.

Merely inserting a silicone implant in a long, loose, hanging breast, absent of fat and glandular tissue, would result in an abnormal appearing breast, because the breast skin and scant breast tissue would override and overhang the implant.

I am ashamed to be seen without my shirt because I always take a kidding about my chest looking like a girl's. I have large breasts like those of a woman. Can I have plastic surgery to make my chest flat? Will the scars show?

Excessive development of male breast tissue is called gynecomastia. This overdeveloped male breast can be safely removed surgically. The surgical procedure entails making an incision in the natural groove or breast fold beneath the breast, undermining the skin leaving the nipple intact, and removing the excess breast tissue and skin. The scars when healed are hidden in the skin folds.

This surgery for gynecomastia, is of great importance to the male who suffers embarrassment and psychological trauma due to his female breast contour. Enlargement of the breast tissue is common in the overweight male, particularly those with endocrine disturbance.

Parents should watch for signs of emotional distress in the teenager who has developed a female-appearing breast. It is at puberty that breast overdevelopment is likely to appear, due to overstimulation of normal hormonal activity. The young male showing these symptoms should be examined for possible medical control of his hormone imbalance, and, where necessary, examined by a plastic surgeon for evaluation for surgical correction of the defect.

Does one feel pressure or extra weight from the inserted breast prosthesis?

Immediately after the operative procedure, some fullness in the chest is felt and some women may experience vague pains for a period of several weeks. After complete healing has taken place, the sensation of fullness disappears as well as any sense of discomfort. The weight of the implants is not felt since they are well supported by the wall of the chest and the overlying breast tissue.

Has there been any evidence of cancer resulting from the insertion of prosthetic material for breast augmentation?

There has most definitely been no occurrence of breast cancer due to insertion of preformed silicone breast implants. Likewise, there have been no cases reported from the insertion of liquid silicone into the breast. Where reports have been made of cancer as a result of the insertion of silicone, liquid or otherwise, into the breast area, the claims have *not* been substantiated by scientific research.

Experiments which caused animals to develop implant carcinogenesis have never been demonstrated in human beings. During fifteen years of exhaustive research, no tumor, benign or malignant, has ever been observed in human tissues that were in direct physical contact with surgically implanted silicone.

**How long is the recovery after
breast augmentation surgery?**

The period of recovery is, conservatively, about three weeks. The sutures are removed within five to seven days and a firm cotton bra is worn to support the breasts. This firm bra is worn also at night for three weeks to one month. There will be normal postoperative swelling for about ten days to two weeks. The suture line will fade and will be barely noticeable after several weeks; however, the scar may remain red for several months. During the recovery period activities are restricted, and the patient must avoid raising the arms, lifting heavy weights, and performing any arduous physical manipulations.

**Where is the incision placed for a
breast implant. Will anyone notice
the scar?**

Only one external surgical incision is made through the skin, and it is hidden under the breast in the mammary fold. The incision is made as short as possible—just long enough to allow the silicone implant to be slipped into place. The silicone implant is selected for size and shape by the surgeon and is placed in a pocket made between the breast tissue and the musculature of the chest wall. The implant usually has an adhesive patch attached to its back surface which adheres to the fibrous tissue covering (fascia) of the muscle of the chest wall.

The closure of the incision is made with a subcuticular suture. This type of suture is one which is placed under the skin edges and the result is a fine hairline scar.

The silicone implant can also be placed under the breast tissue through an incision made in the region of the areola (nipple). The inflatable type of silicone implant is inserted through this type of incision. The areola incision, like the submammary incision, heals well and is even less noticeable than a submammary scar.

If I have silicone implants to enlarge my breasts, do I have to be careful about injuries or pressure on my breasts? Can my breast implants be punctured?

Accidental injuries such as a severe blow to the chest or a crushing blow incurred in an automobile injury can cause a tear or puncture of the breast prosthesis. In these cases, it would be advisable to have the implant immediately removed. The danger of leaving the damaged breast implants would be similar to the action of injected liquid silicone, namely, the gel would travel to surrounding tissue after the covering had been torn apart. If infection to the chest wall should occur following injury, the infection can be more quickly controlled by removing the prosthesis. After the infection has subsided and disappeared, the silicone breast prosthesis can be safely reinserted.

I want to have my breasts enlarged but I plan to have more children. Will I be able to breast-feed my baby?

Future breast-feeding will not be disturbed after augmentation breast surgery. The breast is elevated as a whole from the chest wall at the time of surgery and the silicone breast implant is inserted between the breast tissue and the chest wall.

The lactiferous ducts, which are in the breast tissue and attached to the nipple, are neither exposed nor touched by any surgical instruments in this procedure; therefore, the function of the breast is kept intact and the breast is merely *elevated* from its former position by the silicone implant.

If I have silicone implants inserted to enlarge my breasts, is there a risk of the implants moving out of place?

The breast implant is usually placed in a pocket made by the surgeon under the breast tissue proper and the pocket is made not much larger than the implant. This method of augmentation prevents undue movement of the breast implant. The implant is snug in the pocket without causing any tension on the skin and blood vessels. Further, the back of the implant has a Dacron fixation patch which adheres to the chest wall. In addition, some implants have Dacron fixation patches with a loop, and it is through the loop that the surgeon can place a suture which helps to anchor and prevent rotation of the implant.

Plastic surgeons frequently choose a silicone gel implant without fixation patches and loops. This round implant is the most popular shape chosen by surgeons today because it does not matter if the round prosthesis rotates. The "tear drop" silicone implant, if it be the choice of the surgeon, should have a fixation patch to prevent rotation.

Would anyone who feels my breast after silicone breast augmentation know that I have had surgery?

To the average person palpation of a newly implanted prosthetic breast several weeks after operation will not reveal anything abnormal. This can truly be a woman's secret if she desires to keep it so.

The breasts appear full, erect, and well positioned. To palpation, the breasts are soft but firm, mobile, and elastic. The breasts have a natural appearance in every way and resemble the ideal maiden's breast.

**Could I have any health problems
that would necessitate removal of
silicone breast implants?**

There is little likelihood that a silicone breast implant
need be removed for health reasons, except in the rare
instance where cancer of the breast is the diagnosis. The
cancerous tumor would not be associated with the implant itself, since experimental and clinical evidence
shows no link between silicone implants and malignant
tumors of the breast.

Occasionally a patient may develop an infection at
the point of incision following breast implantation,
postoperatively, or at a much later date. The infection
might be due to a suture remnant that remained in the
region of the incision. When the buried suture is seen, it
is removed and the infection treated with an antibiotic
and hot compresses. Under this circumstance, it would
not be necessary to remove the silicone implant.

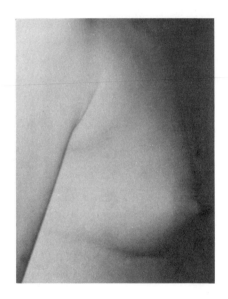 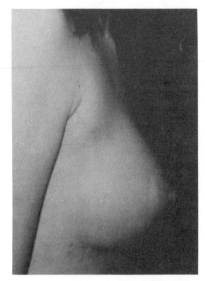

Mammaplasty with silicone implants for breast augmentation

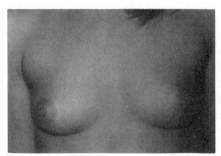 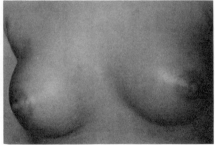

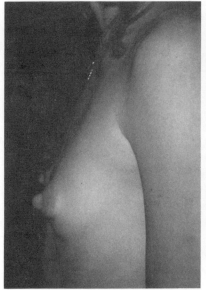 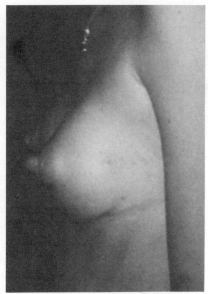

Mammaplasty with silicone implants for breast augmentation

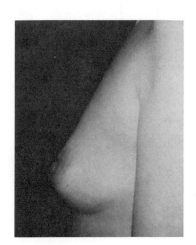 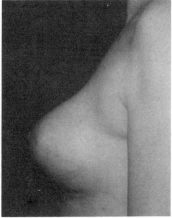

The postoperative picture shows incision line one week after surgery. Incision line will fade and will not be noticed even upon close examination.

Mammaplasty: breast reduction

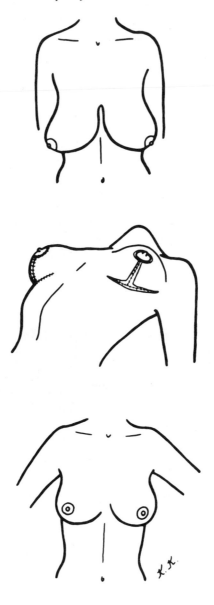

cosmetic body surgery

The human body can be a reservoir of fat that makes a man or woman unattractive, unhealthy, and unhappy. Plumpness, a euphemism for obesity, may have sex appeal in the eyes of some beholders, but in the world of social encounter, the slim, well-proportioned figure attracts more approving glances from the opposite sex. Plastic surgery of the body can come to the rescue of the distressed male or female in many cases of obesity, but, unfortunately, it cannot overcome the poor eating habits of indulgent individuals or the hereditary characteristics of the large proportioned torso.

Pools of fat gather more readily in certain portions of the body—in the female, on the hips, thighs, buttocks, arms, and waist, and in the male, on the waist, buttocks, and back of the neck.

Diet and exercise will go a long way toward helping many overweight people reach an acceptable body figure within the range of normalcy. However, when good and healthful attempts to restore the body to normal proportion fail and the torso shows bulging of skin and rolls of fat as well as sagging muscles, fat, and skin, a consultation with a plastic surgeon is warranted. Help may be available in cosmetic surgery.

Incisions are made into natural folds of the body to

excise excess fat and tighten loose muscles. Operating to eliminate excess fat in areas that provide *no* natural folds and instead require incisions along exposed skin areas becomes more complicated, involving the decision to balance function, exposure of the scars, and aesthetics. Acceptability of the exposed scar that results from cosmetic surgery of the body is a dominating factor in the mutual agreement between surgeon and patient to proceed with surgical body recontouring.

Body surgery that particularly lends itself to good cosmetic results is the abdominal surgery of hyperadiposity or an "apron of fat" so extensive at times that it completely covers the genitalia, causing constant irritation, weeping and itching of the skin in the folds of the apron. The lower abdomen feels heavy and is a source of annoyance and fatigue. Indications for abdominal lipectomy, as discussed here, are those of great necessity, not merely cosmetic indications. Cosmetic indications are vastly important, however, to the person who desires a normal physical appearance. Both men and women who have enlarged abdomens from excess fat find it difficult to choose clothes of good proportion and to attain eye appeal in dress.

When a plastic surgeon examines a person with an excess abdominal fatty apron and has listened to his cries of woe and complaints of physical discomfort, he will be apt to recommend procedures to eliminate any gross deformity. When the surgeon is convinced in his own mind that the patient has done everything possible with dieting, exercise, and medication for weight reduction, and that he has experienced only failure, the surgeon will be inclined to inform the patient of the surgical procedures that could be performed to provide help and relief.

He will explain to the patient where abdominal incisions are placed. The incision might be horizontal in the middle of the abdomen at the level of the navel or at the

level of the hips and pubic hair. This latter site is preferable because of complete absence of a visible scar when
a bikini is worn.

The surgeon will try to save the navel, preferably by
leaving it in place or by excising it and transplanting it
to a normal position.

The removal of abdominal fat and apron is not a
minor surgical procedure, and the patient may be hospitalized for ten days or two weeks. There is also the
possibility of postoperative infection or hemorrhage as
well as complications from general anesthesia. Considerable discomfort in sitting and walking during the
postoperative period is likely. A regime of dieting will
be important following the surgery, since abdominal
hyperadiposity with apron formation can return with
overindulgence in eating.

Fat embolism (fat droplets circulating in the blood
that could enter the lung or brain) can cause pulmonary
and brain complications. The surgeon gives all of this
information to his patient so that each patient is aware
of the possibility of complications and the risks
involved.

The patient will be told to wear abdominal supports
and lower extremities support (support hose) for several
weeks after surgery.

Obviously, it takes a courageous patient to submit
to this functional and cosmetic surgical correction. Both
surgeon and patient do not enter lightly into the agreement. Fortunately, the results of abdominal lipectomies
are usually highly successful and afford the patient great
physical and mental relief. The operation certainly relieves the strain on the heart.

Abdominal lipectomies cost $1,500 to $3,500. The
average fee is probably $2,500.

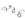

Surgery for buttocks, hips, and thighs is increasing
in popularity because of greater body exposure, the
search for improvement of body contour, and the style

of women's pants which reveal the contour of the hips, buttocks, and thighs. Many people with large hips and thighs who have been disappointed with diets, exercises, and medications seek faster and more positive action with plastic surgery.

Cosmetic hip surgery can be performed for the large, bulging pads of fat by making elliptical incisions of skin and fat at the crest of the hip bone. If the buttock hangs low and is drooping with excess skin and fat, the buttock can be elevated, using the same incision site where skin and fat are removed for the enlarged hips. Additional incisions of skin and excision of fat are made on the lateral (outer) side of the hip for further streamlining; this results in an L-shaped exposed scar. Recontouring the excessively bulging buttock alone requires an incision in the natural fold between buttock and thigh; this scar would be well hidden.

Enlarged thighs with superfluous skin and fat are brought into proper proportions by removing the fat and skin in the region of the groin. Additional incisions on the inner surface of the thigh are used to reduce the superfluous skin and fat on the inner sides of the thighs.

An added problem of aging and obesity is the hanging of excess fat from the arms. In fact, this loose skin appears as a normal sympton of aging even when obesity is absent. The woman who wants to wear a sleeveless dress is frustrated when she observes herself in the mirror.

To correct these drooping deformities of the arms, an elliptical excision of skin and fat is made at the back of the arm. Sometimes this involves the entire length of the arm and sometimes only a portion of the length of the arm. Naturally the major muscles, nerves, and blood vessels of the arm are avoided. Satisfying results from reshaping a flabby arm are attainable. Women who are unhappy about this deformity of aging or obesity should not hesitate to consult a plastic surgeon about correction. A well-placed vertical scar on the inner arm facing toward the body can heal as a fine hairline scar and be inconspicuous, especially if a sleeved dress is worn to cover the evidence of this surgery.

Fees for plastic surgery of the hips are $500 to $1,000. If combined with surgery for drooping buttocks, the fee would be approximately $1,500 to $2,500. Fee range for thigh lift is approximately $1,500 to $2,000. Fees for arm lift are $750 to $1,000.

I am forty-four years old but do not look my age. However, in the last two years my hands have aged tremendously. What can a plastic surgeon do for my protruding veins and tiny wrinkles?

If the wrinkles are numerous enough to cause a severe cosmetic deformity, a surgical technique can be performed for excision of superfluous skin. This procedure tightens the skin of the back of the hands to restore a more youthful appearance. A linear incision is placed along the outer side (small finger side) of the hand. The skin is tightened on this line. A complication of this type of surgery is a temporary limited motion of the hand; also a conspicuous scar may result because of the continuous shifting of the skin due to necessary and normal hand movement.

Droplet silicone injections can be made at intervals under the skin of the back of the hand. It spreads as a film under the skin and obscures the veins from view. Silicone injections hold no dangers when used in this manner, but if, inadvertently, they are injected into a blood vessel of the hand, the silicone could cause an embolism. In this case, a foreign material clot could travel to the heart or brain with the resulting stroke or death. This complication is unlikely to occur when the procedure is performed by a competent surgeon; he always picks up the skin and draws back on the silicone-filled syringe, thus ascertaining immediately that the needle is in or out of a blood vessel. Thus silicone is injected with extreme caution and control. However, at the present time silicone injections are not permitted by the Food and Drug Administration.

Dermal abrasion of the hands can be considered for wrinkling of the hand but the scars that can result destroy every benefit that might be obtained by this technique. (This is in contrast to the beneficial effects of dermal abrasion to the skin of the face.) The skin texture of the hands does not take kindly to the abrasive wheel of dermal abrasion.

Chemical peeling is not suitable for application to the surface of the back of the hand. The texture of the skin is so different from that of the face that again, as with dermal abrasion, it offers more risk than benefit. Chemicals, however, can be applied to individual, small blemishes on the back of the hand. A mild burn will take place and the pigmented areas will dry, scab, and peel off, leaving a much lighter textured area that will blend better with the neighboring skin of the back of the hand.

I dread wearing a short sleeve dress or blouse because of the hanging flesh on my upper arms. I have tried exercises but cannot firm this part of my arms. Can this hanging skin be removed surgically?

Your deformity (bat wing arms) can be corrected with an elliptical incision on the inner surface of the upper arm and removal of the excess skin, subcutaneous tissue, and fat, without disturbing the underlying muscles. The resultant vertical scar, facing toward your body, should not be easily discernible. Wearing a sleeved dress will cover any evidence of this surgery. Following surgery, you may return in about two weeks to routine duties providing you avoid stretching and lifting heavy weights, or moving vigorously in certain sports.

My thighs and buttocks are too heavy
and I am willing to consider plastic
surgery to improve my appearance. But
I would like to know if dieting and
exercise would improve this condition
before I undergo surgery?

Some women can attain success with a program of
weight loss which would reduce their thighs and buttocks and at the same time tighten the local muscles.
Others will lose weight in all parts of the body except
the buttocks and thighs—the area where women normally carry the most fat, especially after menopause.
The older woman whose daily routine keeps her from
normal physical activity is more subject to spreading in
the lower third of the torso. With such women, surgical
procedures are the only method of removing this excess
skin and fat.

An elliptical excision of skin and fat is made from
the outer portion of the thigh, hip, and pelvis, which
raises the buttocks and reduces the size of the thigh.
This is an operation that is not without hazards and is
not recommended except for drastic reasons of health
or appearance. A thorough examination by an internist
and a consultation between him and the surgeon are
good preparations for such surgery.

Why did I form this "apron" of
skin overhanging my abdomen? I feel
I perform the normal amount of
activity of the average adult and
I am not overweight.

Most likely at one time in your life you were extremely
overweight and then went on a "crash" diet. Within a
period of a few weeks you possibly lost a large amount
of weight. The subcutaneous fat that you had was lost,
leaving just skin. The extraneous skin folded upon itself,
forming an "apron." Technically we call this condition
"pendulous abdomen."

Another cause of an apron of abdominal skin is pregnancy; the skin and subcutaneous fat have been stretched due to the pregnancy. The stretched skin and fat, instead of shrinking back into a normal position, form a permanent deformity.

Although a pendulous abdomen is more frequent in women over forty years of age, men too can develop this deformity due to fluctuating obesity and loss of fat from dieting.

The apron of skin can also be associated with hernias or loss of muscle tone following systemic diseases. In these cases the operation for removal of the pendulous apron would involve a repair of the hernia and medical treatment for the systemic disease.

I find my appearance very unattractive due to a pendulous abdomen. I also cannot fit well into fashionable clothes. Besides cosmetic improvement, would I derive any other benefits from plastic abdominal surgery?

Because of the excessive amount of weight and strain on the skeletal system, the pendulous abdomen will cause postural disturbances and put stress on the normal curvature of the spinal column. The unpleasant sensation of heaviness of the torso which frequently inhibits ambulation (walking, running, engagement in sports) is relieved. Limited motion in sexual activity is a frequent accompaniment of the large, pendulous abdomen, and where this occurs, there is a legitimate reason for correction.

Where there are pendulous breasts in addition to a pendulous abdomen, respiration can become more difficult and in time cause strain on the heart.

The folds of the pendulous abdomen are subject to irritation of the skin, with and without ulceration, manifesting itself by itching and weeping of skin ulcers.

After several pregnancies I find the skin of my abdomen flabby and covered

with stretch marks. Can surplus skin
be removed by a plastic surgeon? What
is the surgical procedure?

> The surgeon performing an abdominal lipectomy will
> evaluate how much skin and fat will need to be removed
> to reduce the abdomen to normal proportions for your
> body build. When you are in the hospital, he may have
> you stand up while he outlines the amount of ab-
> dominal excess skin and fatty tissue that can safely be
> removed to include as much of the stretch marks as
> possible.
>
> The incision is usually a horizontal one stretching
> from one hip to the other, dipping down to the center
> to skirt the upper margin of the pubic hairs to partially
> camouflage the scar. It will then fall below the upper
> border of a bikini. The patient is informed that only a
> subtotal removal of stretch marks is possible.
>
> The operation is performed under general anesthesia
> with the patient properly prepared preoperatively.
>
> Postoperatively the patient will be permitted to
> walk for short periods of time the day after surgery. The
> operative dressings will remain in place for about five
> days. There will be some discomfort with sneezing or
> coughing or laughing. An abdominal support will be re-
> quired for several months to insure good healing and
> comfort.

What is the operative procedure to
remove my pendulous abdominal skin?
Will the scars be very obvious?

> The abdominal operation for removal of excessive fat
> and skin is not technically difficult and you can expect
> a reasonably good correction of this deformity. Healing
> is slow and scars are sometimes larger than we would
> hope for. Activity will be restricted for a reasonable
> period to assure good closure of the wound. If umbilical
> (navel) hernia is present and repaired at the same time,
> the convalescence is longer.

Surgeons will always attempt to save the navel (belly button) in abdominal plastic surgery; however, at times this must be sacrificed. Such requirements would be discussed with you prior to surgery.

An abdominal girdle may be advised following surgery. It should be worn for about two months.

The gratifying results of abdominal lipectomy are improved posture, improved body contour, the disappearance of the sensation of "dragging and pulling," and the removal of a constant weight or load from the action of the heart. Cardiologists are beginning to appreciate this fact.

Is there danger to general health in having major surgery for removal of excess skin from the abdomen? What are the risks taken?

The patients who require abdominal lipectomy are frequently those not in the ideal state of health, and they are usually poor surgical risks because of being overweight. A physical examination by the internist and surgeon often reveals high blood pressure, diabetes, and poor general muscle tone. These patients frequently have enlarged hearts and early arteriosclerosis. An evaluation of the patient's medical status is extremely important because of the nature of the surgery. Lipectomy surgery may last several hours under general anesthesia. The operation could be further prolonged because of repair of a possible abdominal hernia. The more prolonged the general anesthesia, the greater is the risk. To insure a safe corrective operation, clearance for surgery should be obtained from the internist, anesthetist, and surgeon.

My thighs are flabby, and dieting and exercise have not improved their appearance. Can I have plastic surgery for surplus skin and fat on my thighs?

Corrective plastic surgery for removal of excess skin and fat of the thighs can be done by excising an elliptical wedge of skin and fat on the outer or inner surface of the thigh or both. The procedure is actually a thigh lift and may also require excision of excess skin in the groin area to obtain a better cosmetic result.

The scars may be visible for some time but will fade after several months. You may not choose to expose your body in a swim suit if the scars do not please you, but the improved way your clothes will fit may be the satisfaction you are seeking, making scars tolerable under the circumstances.

Is it necessary for me to lose my excess weight before having plastic surgery for my loose abdominal skin?

Every surgeon will agree that there are fewer complications with patients who have normal weight for their body height. If you are interested in proper diet and exercise, you can come as close as possible to the ideal surgical patient.

If you have never weighed much less than your present adult weight in spite of attempts to diet and provided that medical clearance is obtainable, you may have the surgery. The procedure may have to be modified in the amount of tissue removed; this must be determined by your surgeon.

Does the fat removed in abdominal plastic surgery tend to return if I regain weight lost in dieting?

Your physician will advise you in maintaining a good nutritional program that will prevent excessive gain in weight. However, the fat that has been surgically removed seldom reconstitutes itself in the body.

What has caused stretch marks on my abdomen? I have had only one pregnancy. If I have plastic surgery to eliminate

them, will they recur with another
pregnancy?

The stretch marks (striae) are caused by an over-extension of the elastic fibers of the skin. The fibers ruptured and the result was a scarring of the surface of the skin. This can happen with just one pregnancy, especially if the abdominal skin has been stretched taut by an unusually large fetus.

Plastic surgery can remove some of these stretch marks by excision of the excess skin containing the stretch marks and bringing the skin edges together. The surgeon attempts to place the incision in a natural fold of the skin and chooses a location where the incision when healed would not be exposed when the patient wears a two-piece bathing suit with bare midriff or a bikini.

If you have another pregnancy there will again be stretching of the elastic fibers of the skin and new striae will appear.

Thigh, hip, and buttock lipectomy

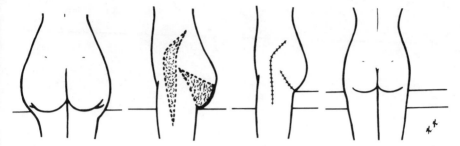

Abdominal lipectomy: removal of fatty apron with incision below bikini line

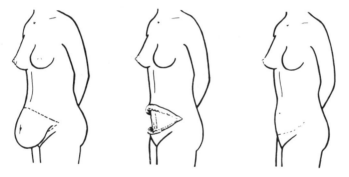

Lipectomy: correction of bat-wing arms

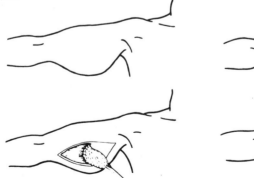
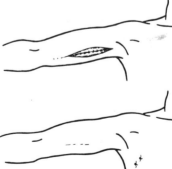

miscellaneous

Many frequently asked questions concerning facial plastic surgery are unclassifiable. But they are important enough to be answered, and we have placed them in this miscellaneous group. Several questions can apply to any surgical specialty, but they are included here because they arise in the minds of patients contemplating plastic surgery. Minor categories, such as surgical tattooing and sex change, are also covered.

Many factors come into play when a patient is discussing cosmetic surgery—fear of pain, concern about finances, chariness about appearing foolish or vain to friends, skepticism about the effectiveness of procedures, depression over personal affairs, and an attempt to use plastic surgery to overcome emotional stress. There are probably many unasked questions that fall into these categories, but experience has proven that the majority of people are concerned about the same or similar matters and characteristically ask the same questions.

Can plastic surgery correct my very thick lips?

There are cosmetic surgical procedures performed for an overabundant lip formation called cheiloplasty. A prominent lip can be due to conditions beyond this feature itself: the jaw position must be noted; dental occlusion is a consideration; and the protrusion or recession of the chin in relation to the normal human profile can be a factor. A "full" lip and prominent mouth are not always undesirable features; in fact, the full, round mouth is symbolic of youth, while the recessed lips are suggestive of aging. By our standards of beauty the most desirable are full lips. And in the history of facial cosmetic adornment there is ample evidence that the lips were the earliest feature to be decorated with color, and the lure of shapely lips was employed to attract the opposite sex by enticing motions.

Among the races, the Negroid lips are distinctive for their tendency toward protrusion and excessive thickness of the vermillion border. However, when the moist, inner lining of the lower lip (the mucous membrane) is visible, there is a cosmetic defect in the average standard appearance of the Negroid lip. While the distinctive appearance of the Negroid lip is accepted by the great majority, there are those who wish to have a more Caucasian-looking appearance, and, for those, plastic surgery has a remedy.

If it has been determined that the chin is the deformity causing the unaesthetic lip formation, a mentoplasty for chin correction is performed, as a primary procedure. The surgeon then awaits the resulting effect before going on to a second operation for the lips.

I have always admired dimples and wondered if I could have these made by plastic surgery?

Dimples in the cheeks can be made by plastic surgery. The plastic surgeon will use a six to eight millimeter trephine (skin punch) for making a dimple. He anesthetizes the inside of the cheek and will remove a plug of tissue from inside of the mouth at the point where the dimple is to appear on the exterior surface of the face. After removing the plug, the surgeon closes the wound with one or two sutures, grasping the base of the skin and "dimpling" it inward. The skin of the face is now pulled in the direction of the oral cavity, thus forming a "dimple."

Is it true that all cosmetic surgeons demand payment in cash, in full, and in advance?

It is true that cosmetic plastic surgeons have an office policy of having their secretary discuss the fee arrangement with the patient, explaining that payment in full will be expected several weeks in advance of the surgical date. *Method* of payment (check, cash, money order) is the choice of the patient.

The reason for this fee payment in advance is to insure a firm, well-planned hospital and surgeon's schedule. In most major cities, hospital bed space is at a premium, as is operating room time. The patient must bear in mind that his surgery is *elective,* rather than necessary for health. The bulk of hospital surgery is performed for life-saving reasons and naturally takes precedent over elective surgery. The hospital operating room supervisor will not contend long with surgeons who book cases and cancel them close to the day of surgery. It is a loss of critical and valuable time to the hospital. The surgeon finds it an unnecessary loss of his time since he has allotted this time (usually many hours) for the patient. The patient who has paid his fee in advance has assured the surgeon and, through him, the hospital, that he is financially responsible and has made up his mind to undergo the surgery. An avoidance of unwarranted ill feeling between patient and surgeon and surgeon and hospital is accomplished by prepayment.

Can I have my eyebrows lifted? Will a scar be seen?

Cosmetic eyelid surgery includes the technique of lifting a part or the entire eyebrow. Lifting the temporal ends of the eyebrows gives them an "upswept" appearance.

This curving upward of the brow is accepted in our culture as exotic and as suggestive of "sex appeal." Regardless of its cultural connotation, it also provides a smoother upper eyelid, eliminating many wrinkles of the upper lid and giving a broader base for the glamorous cosmetics of the day.

The scar from the incision is often the deterrent to its more popular acceptance as a routine procedure by facial and ophthalmic plastic surgeons. The incision above the normal eyebrow line hardly ever falls into a natural fold like that of the eyelid itself; in fact it should be made just within the eyebrow hairline. Some eyebrows have generous growth of hair for additional disguise of the scar's presence.

Facial makeup is an excellent aid in covering the scar, but the scar is there, and you may be the unlucky person on whom the scar is more evident than on another. Men cannot cover the scar with makeup without being subjected to ridicule. Therefore, no facial surgeon will perform an eyebrow lift as a routine procedure in cosmetic eyelid surgery without discussing the possibility of a permanent scar in this area.

I have very few eyelashes. Can this be corrected by plastic surgery?

Although upper eyelids normally contain a supply of lashes numbering 150-200 growing in two or three rows, you obviously have a less abundant growth. However, hair transplantation is seldom performed successfully below the scalp. This is not to say that hair transplants are not attempted in unusual areas as along the margin of the upper eyelid to enrich the eyelash line. In fact, the Japanese surgeons have been doing this for years by making an incision just above the upper eyelashes and transplanting hair from the scalp into that incision. The patient, however, is warned that he has to trim the growth of this new hair frequently to match the length of his own lashes. If and when there is some alteration in the direction of growth of these new lashes the surgeon can remove the transplant.

Other unusual areas of transplantation are the male upper lip where he cannot grow a mustache or his chin for a desired goatee when he finds his natural growth too sparse. However, such esoteric applications of the hair transplantation technique have not come into common usage in this country.

Cosmetologists apply individual eyelashes for the woman who desires a full-looking fringe of eyelashes. With due care this application of lashes remains in place for three to four weeks before they gradually fall out one by one, at which time they can be successfully reapplied. This particular beauty care, like hair tinting and hair setting, has to be renewed periodically.

I have no eyebrows. Can a plastic surgeon create an eyebrow by transplanting hair?

It is conceivable that hair transplantation could be employed on the person devoid of eyebrows. There are vital factors to be considered before attempting this procedure: the texture and quality of the hair to be transplanted (usually from the scalp); the direction of the growth of the hair (the eyebrow pattern is distinctly nasal to temporal in direction of growth); the feasibility of frequent trimming to maintain a normal brow line; and the estimated period of healing time for the transplants. The possibility of failure is real and the scars that would remain from individual or strip grafts could be a serious cosmetic deformity.

What surgical feat of facial plastic surgery is most satisfying to the patient?

In our experience and that of many other plastic surgeons, the restoration of the more youthful appearance of the neck brings the greatest joy to the greatest number. Women in tears and men close to tears smile blissfully when they no longer see the loose, hanging flesh beneath the chin and the heavy creases of the neck after a surgical face and neck lift.

The age of the patient is a factor in the choice of surgery that gives him the most gratification. The younger person, first troubled by the loose skin or fatty bags around the eyelids, may find corrective eyelid surgery the source of much happiness. But we opt for the devastated middle-aged patient who has suddenly "turned old overnight" and is in despair over the jowls and wattles in the lower jaw and neck.

I have a criminal record and have a long association with "undesirable" people. Can I have my facial features changed radically enough so that I would not be recognized by my former associates?

Your facial features are not the only means of identifying you. You are recognized by your hair, your skin color, your eyes, your teeth, the inflection of your voice, your manner of speech, your height, your body shape and weight, and many habits and gestures unique to you. Changing your nose by rhinoplasty, or ears by otoplasty, or skin condition of face and eyes by face lift and blepharoplasty will make some changes in your general appearance but hardly enough to make you unidentifiable.

If you have served your debt to society for crimes committed and you desire to become a responsible citizen by gainful employment and establishing beneficial social contacts, you can rightly consider any facial plastic surgery which will improve your appearance and elevate your self-esteem. You are certainly entitled to correct any deformities, congenital (by birth) or acquired, as well as to seek surgery for restoration of a more youthful look. Any plastic surgery that will give you confidence in yourself is most imperative for your successful rehabilitation.

**If I do not want anyone to know I am
in the hospital, can I enter under an
assumed name?**

Legal arrangements can be made for your entering a hospital under an assumed name. Your lawyer should be consulted to prepare the way. He will speak with the hospital administrator as your legal representative. He will also speak with the insurance company who carries your hospitalization so that an alias will be acceptable to them and the name agreed upon in advance. Since the purpose is to keep your own identity from public knowledge, the matter would have to be handled ethically, legally, and discreetly; hence the need for legal advice and representation.

**Will you do cosmetic surgery on me
even though I am under legal age?**

Neither facial plastic surgeons nor general surgeons will perform surgery on anyone under legal age without written permission from parent or guardian.

In rare circumstances where serious conflict of interest between child and parents was involved, legal aid was sought for a court order permitting surgery to be performed on a person under legal age.

In some states legal responsibility is recognized in the individual who, although under legal age, is married and gainfully employed in self-support or as head of household support. A lawyer could clarify your position in this regard.

**Will hormone pills halt some of the
natural aging process of the skin?**

Hormone medication is prescribed by many physicians to maintain the normal endocrinological balance in the human body. The body in its younger years has a more ideal chemical balance, with all glands and body organs nourishing the body. The skin, like other beneficiaries of this well-organized feeding system, is soft and supple. When this complicated mechanism that keeps us youthfully beautiful begins to misfire, or fail completely, our bodies are the unhappy, unfortunate victims. Hormone pills are often prescribed to recrank the rusty machinery and get the wheels rolling again to resume delivery of, or increase, hormonal activity. Logically, this might indicate that these hormones will halt the natural aging process of the skin, but there is no firm proof that the skin will benefit by better endocrinological balance in the postmenopausal age. However, if hormones are prescribed by a physician, he has concluded from examination and laboratory verification that you need them for essential body function. Maintaining physical good health is necessary and beneficial to all segments of the body, the skin is no exception. Although there is no medication to tighten flabby muscles and replenish lost fat cushioning under the skin, hormones, vitamins, and minerals are credited with maintaining but not restoring a healthy skin.

Why cannot a surgeon guarantee the results of surgery?

The practice of medicine involves art and science. It is impossible, therefore, for any physician or surgeon to predict unerringly, let alone guarantee, the results of any medical treatment or surgical procedure he performs. The surgeon's experience and knowledge afford him a certain degree of predictability concerning results of operations he performs. Statistics accumulated by operating surgeons and case histories that have been written in medical journals add to the knowledge of results obtainable for the majority of surgical procedures. Nature is full of the wonders of healing, but nature can display a fickleness that defies all logic, and, whereas most patients will obtain a beautiful surgical result, a few who undergo the identical surgery will not obtain the optimal result. The chemical processes of the human body control healing in their own unique way. No one in this world is a duplicate of you.

How can I determine if my insurance
policy will provide medical and surgical
coverage for plastic surgery?

Operations performed to correct or lessen deformities
due to congenital defects or injury are, as a general rule
of medical and surgical indemnity, covered by insurance
plans. However, since every insurance company has its
own contract form, this contract must be the determining factor in the decision on the part of the insurance
company to make payment for surgical claims. Many
insurance companies have exclusion clauses in their
policies specifically disallowing indemnity for cosmetic
plastic surgery.

Discuss the cost of surgery with your surgeon, since
plastic surgeons require payment in advance for cosmetic surgery. Every plastic surgeon's office will have a
staff member assist you in making claims for reimburse-
ment and filling out all necessary forms. However, the
plastic surgeon cannot assure you that you will collect
benefits for surgery with your particular insurance
policy.

Why am I unable to obtain a quotation
of a surgical fee on the telephone?

An evaluation of your surgical requirements cannot be
estimated without an examination by the surgical specialist who would be performing the operation. You may
feel certain that you know exactly what you want and
need and can describe this accurately to the surgeon on
the telephone, but you are not in the position to see
yourself as the surgeon sees you. Nor can you judge how
he would plan the correction of your cosmetic problem.

Can I have facial plastic surgery if I
am pregnant?

The pregnant patient would be wiser not to seek an
elective plastic surgical procedure. Every operation
creates some stress that varies in its effects on patients
with different nervous systems. Drugs administered pre-

operatively, operatively, and postoperatively, by mouth and by injection, may affect the pregnancy.

Have rejuvenation clinics anything to offer me as an adjunct to facial plastic surgery?

The pampered rich have long enjoyed the mixed blessings of affording themselves the luxury of special "rejuvenation" treatments in European spas, and they have paid well for this pampering. The clinics in Switzerland and Roumania, for example, have received and treated famous personalities who attest to their restored vigor and good looks after "secret formula" injections and oral medications. In the last few years the "secret formulae" have gone the way of such miracle drugs supposedly known only to the administering physician; they have been revealed to the medical profession and they have been published extensively throughout world journals. Essentially the "restorative" drug is a combination of procaine and high vitamin dosage injected on a controlled basis. Its effect is sometimes multiplied by an oral administration of high dosages of vitamins, particularly, vitamin B-12.

Procaine as commonly administered in the United States is a drug used by surgeons for achieving local anesthesia. It appears that the drug, as prepared and used in Europe intravenously, is different from ours and hence has a different effect. There is no firm scientific evidence for this.

As employed by "Fountain of Youth" clinics, the drug affects the nervous system by combining relaxation with exhilaration, which results in a slightly euphoric sensation. The continued regimen of highly potent vitamin intake provides the aging body with nutrients it is often lacking due to a lifestyle of poor nourishment, overindulgence, lack of sufficient sleep, sporadic, if any, healthful physical activity in the form of sports or exercise, and other of our living habits that destroy us after forty. Apparently, then, the rejuvenation clinics appear to make some sense. However, this therapy has questionable results. Placenta injections for the purpose of rejuvenation by highly touted authorities abroad is frowned upon by the American medical profession because of its dangerous possibilities. Despite it, for some individuals, the psychological and physical assistance of rejuvenation treatment becomes their routine yearly vacation.

Can photographs taken of me pre- and postoperatively be used for display without my permission?

Photographs taken of a patient before and after cosmetic surgery have a well-established protection of medical privacy and cannot be displayed without the patient's permission. However, most patients interested in the progress of cosmetic surgery and the furthering of its attainments are most accommodating when these photographs are to be used in lecturing, writing scientific articles, or persuading fearful patients that good results are commonly achieved.

Permission for display of your photographs is granted by your signing a release form.

I have discussed my desire for a change of sex from male to female with a psychiatrist. I want to know if plastic surgery can assist me in this transformation?

Plastic surgery for sex change is being performed in many large cities of the world. New York, Baltimore, Los Angeles, Paris, and London are only some of the cities where this surgery can be obtained.

The transformation of male to female would probably entail your having breast augmentation with gel-filled silicone implants for a more female looking body contour. The surgery is performed under general or local anesthesia.

Facial features would be made more feminine by performing a rhinoplasty to achieve a more delicate looking nose. The bony structure of the eyebrow area is prominent in males and can be reduced in size. This is accomplished by making an incision in the region of the eyebrow and shaving away some of the bony prominence.

Your neck can be made more female by reduction of the masculine "Adam's apple" (thyroid cartilage of larynx or voice box). An incision is made above the voice box and the prominence of the thyroid cartilage is shaved away without disturbing the function of the vocal cords.

The masculine hair and sweat glands of the armpits can be removed by making a small incision under the armpits and undermining all the skin of the armpits and then using a sharp curette on the undersurface of the skin to peel off the hair follicles and roots and, in addition, the sweat glands.

Facial hair can be eliminated by the same procedure—by making incisions in front of the ear and behind the ear, undermining the skin in the region of the hair growth in the manner of a face lift, and sweeping the undersurface of the skin with a curette to destroy the hair follicles.

Since the male figure is usually slim-hipped, surgery can be performed with the use of silicone implants to round out the buttocks.

After the above surgery is accomplished and the patient is desirous of complete physical sex change, the male genitalia can be surgically reconstructed to simulate female genitalia. This is a special and complex type of reconstructive surgery.

Several friends have asked me how they might overcome their embarrassment about seeking information and advice concerning cosmetic plastic surgery.

**Is there any way to handle
this reluctance?**

The person who desires cosmetic improvement through plastic surgery but who is reluctant to seek professional advice is usually inhibited by feelings of fright of the contemplated surgery or narcissistic thoughts. Both inhibitions are understandable under the circumstances but not warranted.

Fright is easily overcome by the assurance that there is no pain suffered during or after surgery due to the effective medications employed by surgeons. Narcissism, or concern with one's physical appearance, is a normal human trait manifested by mankind through the centuries in varying modes of dress and adornment, use of male and female cosmetics and beauty-enhancing products, control of diet for body weight, ingestion and injection of vitamins, hormones, and other health maintenance drugs, use of fragrances and skin conditioners, even behavioral mannerisms. The realm of self-improvement is a never-ending, ever-changing, always fascinating source of challenge to the bestower of human beauty and the recipient of his talent and originality.

The person desiring cosmetic plastic surgery should summon up his resources of initiative to combine with his motivation for physical improvement and face the truth about himself. The patient with a healthy attitude toward cosmetic surgery will accept its benefits willingly and happily. The plastic surgeon will help him acquire this approach during the consultation by providing the information to allay fears, explaining the goals and limitations of cosmetic surgery, encouraging an honest appraisal of the patient's physical shortcomings, and estimating the expectations of cosmetic improvement through surgery.

**My face has a "dishpan" shape with
my nose and cheeks looking caved in.**

**Can plastic surgery reshape the bones
of my face?**

The recontouring of your face is a major plastic surgical operation that is performed by highly trained and skilled reconstructive plastic surgeons. The technique entails making an incision across the skull from one ear to the other. This incision line will be made behind the hairline and will be well hidden by your hair when it grows over the healed scar line. The skin of the face is separated from the facial bones. The facial bones are then cut across the brow, down along the temples, and to the back of the upper jaw. What has been accomplished at this point is a detachment of the upper portion of the facial bones. Then the surgeon actually pulls the facial bones forward to restore the normal facial contour. The sections of facial bones are now attached to each other by drilling holes in the bones and wiring the bones together, thereby fixing them in their normal position. Missing critical sections of bone needed to maintain the new facial contour are supplied by bone grafts from other portions of the patient's body (hips, ribs). The skin is replaced over the new facial skeletal structure.

**I have lost my ability to function
sexually as a male and want to know if
plastic surgery can help me.**

Male sexual dysfunction due to the inability to have a normal erection during sexual relations can be treated surgically with a silicone implant into the penis. The disturbing feature of this implant is the permanent rigidity of the penis. Before making a decision in favor of surgery your plastic surgeon may want endocrinological and psychiatric clearance.

**Would correcting my receding chin help
me to correct my bite? My dentist says
that my bite is bad and needs to be**

corrected by dental surgery to prevent
my teeth from wearing down.

The dental surgeon has techniques for correcting a poor
bite (malocclusion) that is wearing down teeth. The
receding jaw causing the facial deformity requires intricate surgery combining the skills of the dental surgeon
and the plastic reconstructive surgeon.

A portion of the lower jaw will be cut to allow the
anterior section to be slid forward. Bone transplants and
metal plates may be needed to add to the reconstruction
of the lower jaw to achieve the proper cosmetic proportion and rigidity. With the aid of an orthodontist, the
upper teeth are wired to the lower teeth for immobiliza-
tion of several weeks during the healing period.

The improvement accomplished in correcting your
receding chin will be of considerable assistance in your
bite adjustment.

I have a receding chin that gives me a
very unattractive profile. My dentist
says there is nothing wrong with my
teeth alignment. Can plastic surgery
correct this condition?

A receding chin, with a normal bite, is lacking sufficient
bone structure for normal contour. It is a feature of the
face that is most easily corrected by the implantation of
a section of bone, cartilage, or silicone. The silicone
implant is used by most plastic surgeons today because
of the ease with which it is obtained and shaped to fill
out the deformity. As a foreign material implant, it is
least likely to cause reaction and be rejected by the
body.

Implantation of the silicone is made through an incision placed under the chin where it is not seen when
healed. The procedure is one performed frequently in
conjunction with rhinoplasty because many patients
who have large, deformed noses have some chin reces-

sion. Correcting the nasal deformity by *decreasing* the protrusion of the nasal bridge and *increasing* the protrusion of the chin achieves a most harmonious profile.

How safe is surgical tattooing to cover birthmarks of the face and neck? I am considering this procedure in place of plastic surgery.

Tattooing is safe if performed by medical personnel who use the appropriate sterility and mixture of pigments. Covering the birthmarks and port wine stains by tattooing, a technique based on punctures of the skin and the introduction of pigment, is a helpful adjunct in the cosmetic surgical field. The process can be slow and tedious, and the results not always satisfactory for large areas involved, but this may be the only acceptable course of treatment for some patients.

My young teenage daughter has a protruding jaw. She is now fourteen years of age. What is the correct age for plastic surgery for a protruding jaw?

A girl of fourteen is ready for surgery if she has attained full growth and stature and is in good health. A young person must be well advised about the long postoperative healing period, during which time her teeth are wired for immobility for at least four weeks. She would be on a liquid diet during this period of time.

What is the surgical fee to correct protruding jaw?

There will probably be more than one bill for this surgical technique since there will be more than one surgeon involved. You will receive a bill from the orthodontist who will wire your teeth before surgery and will do additional wiring and adjustment during and after your surgery. You will receive a bill from the plastic surgeon; and if there is an assistant dental oral surgeon, he will present his bill. The plastic surgical portion of the fee will be approximately $1,800 to $2,500. The assistant dental oral surgeon will possibly bill for a fee amounting to about 20 percent of the plastic surgeon's fee. The orthodontist will usually present his fee separately and will advise you of the amount when you are ready to have your preoperative preparation for surgery.

I have heard that some people go abroad for plastic surgery. Why do they choose a foreign country for their surgery?

There are many well trained plastic surgeons in other countries and a patient may choose to go to one of these surgeons because of his world-renown. There could be strictly personal reasons for a patient to choose a foreign plastic surgeon: to avoid unwanted publicity, to be out of notice by friends or relatives, or to have surgery at a more reasonable price in a country where the standard of living makes fees lower than in the United States.

Does altitude or climate have any influence on the condition of the skin, halting or increasing the aging process?

To some limited degree both altitude and humidity or lack of humidity have a bearing on the condition of the skin. High altitude with its accompanying rarified dry air contributes none of the needed moisture to skin. On the contrary it tends to deprive the skin of necessary moisture and increases the aging process, despite the image of agelessness in Shangri-La, high in the Himalayas. In this paradise, it was the idyllic life free of anxiety, not the climate, that halted aging.

Where dry air is accompanied by winds, this battering of the skin adds to wear and tear. Add to that the peppering of the complexion by sand carried on desert winds, and you can well understand that the Sahara, or any desert existence, should not beckon the man or woman who wants to preserve a fine skin.

England, with its cool climate and frequent rain, takes credit for the lovely complexion of English ladies. For that matter, the eastern United States with temperate climate and relatively high year-round humidity would offer an almost equally favorable condition for the moisture-hungry aging skin. If this were the only factor involved in skin care, we could recommend someone to live in a temperate, relatively humid climate with expectation that aging of the skin would be slowed down. But with dirt, smog, and a frenetic way of life imposed upon us, all benefits of climate fade away.

If you live in a hot, dry climate, cover up and feed the skin with moisturizers. If you live in an area with favorable climatic conditions, add to your good fortune with peace of mind and a healthful diet; your visit to a facial plastic surgeon will surely be delayed several years.

Can plastic surgery do anything to reduce the pain, restore the mobility, and help me to regain the shape of my hands which are disfigured from rheumatoid arthritis?

Deformity of the hands due to osteoarthritis and rheumatoid arthritis involves not only the joints but also the ligaments, capsule, and tendons. If surgical correction is needed tendon and ligament reconstruction along with joint reconstruction with the use of silicone implant can be done. The patient accepted for this cosmetic and functional surgery is one whose hands and wrists are painful and whose joints are partly destroyed and dislocated with loss of function. There is no limitation in age. The surgery is made possible because of the remarkable method of performing total joint replacement with silicone implants.

Flexible joint silicone implants help 90 percent of these afflicted people. Research on the use of silicone implants for the last ten years reveals that the results have been satisfactory cosmetically and functionally and afford relief from pain.

Patients who have total joint reconstruction with silicone implants are informed that they have a chronic recurrent condition, that the disease is progressive, and that while one joint has been repaired and is now functioning well, a neighboring joint can become arthritic.

Patients who are going to have this surgery must be in good physical condition and have an adequate amount of bone left in the region of the joint and good normal skin for covering. Also there must not be more than a few finger joints involved with the disease.

*Mentoplasty: correction of receding
chin with silicone implant*

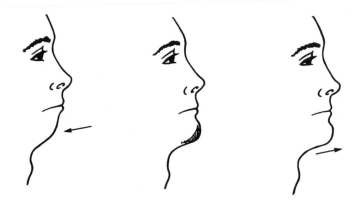

glossary

Abdominoplasty: Plastic surgery of the abdominal wall

Acne: A common, usually chronic, inflammatory disease of the oil glands of the skin, occurring mostly about the face, chest, and back

Ala: Outer wall of each nostril consisting of skin and cartilage

Adipose: Fatty

Analgesia: Insensibility to pain without loss of consciousness

Analgesic: An agent for producing analgesia

Anesthesia: A condition of insensibility to touch or pain

Anterior: Situated before or in front of

Antihelix: The curved ridge of the external ear just below the helix *(q.v.)*

Antisepsis: Use of chemicals to maintain sterility

Areola: The pigmented ring surrounding the breast nipple

Asepsis: Maintenance of sterility by exclusion of microörganisms

b

c

Auricle: The outer expanded portion of the external ear; the pinna *(adj.:* auricular)

Axilla: The armpit

Biopsy: Excision, during life, of a fragment or piece of a new growth to establish the diagnosis by microscopic examination

Blepharoplasty: Plastic surgery of the eyelids

Canthus: The corner of each side of the eye where the upper and lower lids meet

Carcinoma: A malignant tumor

Carcinogenic: Having the property of producing a malignant tumor

Cartilage: A translucent elastic tissue comprising part of the skeleton; gristle *(adj:* cartilaginous)

Cervical: Pertaining to the neck

Cheiloplasty: Plastic reconstruction of lips

Chemosurgery: The surgical application of chemical cauterants to the skin

Chloasma: Patches of dark pigment in the skin

Cilia: Eyelashes

Clavicle: The collarbone

Cleft lip: Harelip

Coagulation: The process of clotting

Collagen: A gelatinlike protein that forms the chief constituent of the fibrils of bone and connective tissue *(adj.:* collagenous)

Columella: The fleshy column separating the nostrils

Congenital: Existing at birth

Conjunctiva: The mucous membrane covering the anterior portion of the globe of the eye and inner aspects of the lid

Crus: Either of two limbs of the antihelix of the ear

Cutaneous: Pertaining to the skin

d

Derma-, dermo-: A combining form meaning skin

Dermabrasion: Surgical abrasion (sanding) of the skin

Dermatitis: An inflammation of the skin

Dermatology: Science and treatment of the skin

Dermis: The layer of skin between the epidermis and the subcutaneous tissue

Dorsum: The back or posterior surface of a part

Dyscrasia: Abnormal composition of the blood

Dysfunction: Impairment of the functioning of an organ

e

Ecchymosis: Black and blue discoloration due to blood in the subcutaneous tissues

Ectropion: Eversion or turning out of a part, especially of an eyelid or lip

Edema: Excessive accumulation of fluid in the tissue spaces; swelling

Endocrine: Any of the ductless glands whose secretions pass directly into the blood stream

Engorged: Swollen with fluids

Entropion: Inversion or turning in of a part, especially of an eyelid or lip

Epicanthus: A congenital anomaly in which a fold of skin covers the inner canthus *(q.v.)*

Epidermis: The outer layer of skin

Epithelium: A cellular lining of a surface or cavity

Estrogen: Female sex hormone

Excise: To cut out

Extravasation: The escape of fluids into the surrounding tissue

f

Fascia: A layer of connective tissue sheathing or supporting the muscles, nerves, and blood vessels

Fibril: A component filament of a fiber; a small thread

Fibrosis: Excess growth of white fibrous connective tissue (scarring)

Flap: A partially detached portion of skin and tissue used as a graft. The flap is transferred on a pedicle and carries its own blood supply from the donor site

g

Glabella: The area of the frontal bone between the eyebrows

Graft: A portion of tissue to replace a defect in the body

Gynoplasty: Plastic surgery of the female reproductive organs

h

Helix: The rounded, convex margin of the external ear

Hemangioma: A benign tumor made up of newly formed blood vessels

Hematoma: A localized blood collection within the tissues

Hemoglobin: The reddish pigment of the blood

Hemostasis: Arrest of blood flow

Hypertrophy: Enlargement or overgrowth due to increase in size of cells

i

Implant: Nonviable material placed beneath the skin to fill a defect in the body, such as silicone

Incise: To cut

Inferior: Lower

k

Keloid: A fibrous overgrowth of scar tissue

Keratin: An albuminoid forming the chemical base of epidermal tissues

Keratosis: A disease of the skin characterized by overgrowth of the horny layers

l

Labial: Pertaining to the lips

Larynx: The organ of voice

Lentigo: A freckle

Lingual: Pertaining to the tongue

Lipectomy: Excision of fatty tissue
Lipoma: A fatty growth

m

Malocclusion: Any deviation from normal occlusion of the teeth

Mammaplasty: Plastic surgery of the breast

Mandible: The lower jawbone

Mastectomy: Excision of the breast

Maxilla: The upper jawbone

Melanin: The dark pigment of the skin

Melanoma: A tumor made up of melanin pigmented cells

Meloplasty: Plastic surgery of the cheek

Mental: Pertaining to the chin (mentum)

Mentoplasty: Plastic surgery of the chin

Mucosa: A mucous membrane

n

Nasolabial: Pertaining to the nose and lip

Necrosis: Death of an area of tissue

Nevus: Pigmented lesion. *See* Melanoma

o

Obesity: An excess of accumulation of fat in the body

Occipital: Pertaining to the back of the head

Occlusion: The efficient meeting of the upper and lower teeth

Orbit: The bony cavity containing the eye

Otoplasty: Plastic surgery of the ear

p

Palpation: Examination with hand

Palpebral: Pertaining to the eyelid

Pharynx: The tube which joins the oral cavity to the esophagus

Plaque: A patch or flat area

Posterior: Situated behind or at the back of

Preauricular: Situated in front of the ear

Prosthesis: An artificial substitute for a missing part of the body

Ptosis: Abnormal depression or drooping

Ptotic: Pertaining to or affected with ptosis

Pulmonary: Pertaining to the lungs

r

Resect: To remove surgically by cutting

Rhinoplasty: Plastic surgery of the nose

Rhytidectomy: Plastic surgery to remove wrinkles, sags, and folds of the face; a face lift

S

Sebaceous: Pertaining to sebum *(q.v.)*

Seborrhea: A functional disease of the sebaceous glands

Sebum: The oily secretion of the sebaceous glands

Septum: A partition between two spaces of cavities, particularly in the nose *(pl.: septa)*

Sloughing: A mass of dead tissue cast out

Striae: Streaks or stripes

Subconjunctival: Situated beneath the mucous membrane covering the anterior portion of the globe of the eye

Subcutaneous: Beneath the skin

Subcuticular: In or under the skin

Submental: Under the chin

t

Transverse: Crosswise; at right angles to the longitudinal axis of the body

Turbinates: Bones or lateral wall of nasal passages

v

Vascular, vaso-: Pertaining to the blood vessels

Venous: Pertaining to the veins

Vermilion: The pigmented border of the lips

z

Zygoma: The cheek bone

index

a

242

CONSULTATION WITH A PLASTIC SURGEON

Breast augmentation, cont.
  removing sutures after, 190
  risks in, 182, 183, 185, 191
  scars from, 191
  by silicone implant, 181, 183, 184-85,
      187, 189-90, 192, 221
  swelling and discoloration after, 183,
      190
  surgical techniques for, 181, 182-83,
      187-88, 190-91
Breast, development of female, 180-81
Breast prothesis. *See* Silicone
    implant
Breast reconstruction (after amputation),
    184, 185-87
  fee for, 187
  research in, 169, 187
  with radical mastectomy, 187
Breast reduction
  for females (mammaplasty), 181, 235
  for males (gynecoplasty), 181, 188-89
  and the nipple, 181
  reasons for, 181, 189
  surgical techniques for, 181, 188-89
Breast surgery. *See* Breast augmentation;
    Breast reconstruction; Breast
    reduction
Brevitol, 28
Bufferin, 37
Burns, 126

C

Chemical skin peeling (chemosurgery),
    9, 16, 22, 26, 108, 110, 111, 124,
    129, 132, 135-48, 172, 202, 232
  adhesive taping after, 138, 147-48
  aftercare for, 139, 148
  anesthesia for, 146
  chemical action of, 135-36, 137, 146
  chemical choice for, 135, 145, 146-47
  correction of, 141, 148
  defects not corrected by, 141, 145
  discomforts and pain of, 137, 138, 146
  drugs used with, 137, 145-46
  effectiveness of, 135, 138, 141-42,

d

e

f

g

h

i

j

k

l

m

n

O

r

s

t

About the Authors

The authors are founders and directors of the New York Facial Plastic Reconstructive Surgery Group, New York City, and founder-members of the International Academy of Cosmetic Plastic Surgery, Geneva, Switzerland.

Dr. Dicker has lectured widely on plastic surgery in America and in foreign countries, including Japan, Russia, South Africa, Ethiopia, Greece, and Iran.

Dr. Syracuse was a member of the first class in America to study cosmetic plastic surgery. Later he joined Dr. Samuel Fomon, another pioneer, who founded the first school of plastic surgery. He taught here for twenty years.

Dr. Syracuse has also lectured abroad on facial surgery—in Japan, Russia, Austria, Italy, and Rumania. With Dr. Fomon, he was co-author of numerous articles on plastic surgery that appeared in professional journals, including *Archives of Otolaryngology* (American Medical Association) and *Ear, Nose and Throat Monthly.*